HOW TO DETOXIFY YOUR LIFE NATURALLY

Sri Regine Lherisson-Bey

Library of Congress Cataloging-in-Publication Data:
Control number: 1-2032431341
ISBN Number: 978-0-9895717-1-5
HOW TO DETOXIFY YOUR LIFE NATURALLY

5th Edition

US Library of Congress copyright.
Common Law copyright and UCC 1-103 copyright and trademark; UCC 3-503
All rights, liberties, and remedies reserved with prejudice. Non-assumpsit.

Printed in the United States of America.

TABLE OF CONTENTS

"The new science of epigenetics reveals that environmental information controls our genes, health and behavior. In humans, the composition of the blood represents those "controlling" factors. In addition to the neurotransmitters from the brain, the blood's influence is mediated by our nutrition and environmental toxins. In **HOW TO DETOXIFY YOUR LIFE NATURALLY**, Sri Regine Lherisson-Bey provides an important guide to clearing your system of toxins and enhancing your health. This is a definite guide for those seeking a life of health and love."

Bruce H. Lipton, Ph.D.
Cell biologist and best selling author of *The Biology of Belief*

Biography

Bruce H. Lipton, PhD is an internationally recognized leader in bridging science and spirit. Stem cell biologist, bestselling author of The Biology of Belief and recipient of the 2009 Goi Peace Award, he has been a guest speaker on hundreds of TV and radio shows, as well as keynote presenter for national and international conferences.

Dr. Lipton began his scientific career as a cell biologist. He received his Ph.D. Degree from the University of Virginia at Charlottesville before joining the Department of Anatomy at the University of Wisconsin's School of Medicine in 1973. Dr. Lipton's research on muscular dystrophy, studies employing cloned human stem cells, focused upon the molecular mechanisms controlling cell behavior. An experimental tissue transplantation technique developed by Dr. Lipton and colleague Dr. Ed Schultz and published in the journal Science was subsequently employed as a novel form of human genetic engineering.

In 1982, Dr. Lipton began examining the principles of quantum physics and how they might be integrated into his understanding of the cell's information processing systems. He produced breakthrough studies on the cell membrane, which revealed that this outer layer of the cell was an organic homologue of a computer chip, the cell's equivalent of a brain. His research at Stanford University's School of Medicine, between 1987 and 1992, revealed that the environment, operating through the membrane, controlled the behavior and physiology of the cell, turning genes on and off. His discoveries, which ran counter to the established scientific view that life is controlled by the genes, presaged one of today's most important fields of study, the science of epigenetics. Two major scientific publications derived from these studies defined the molecular pathways connecting the mind and body. Many subsequent papers by other researchers have since validated his concepts and ideas.

v

*This book is dedicated to
the Universe
and all the evolving life forms that it is a host to.*

In acknowledgement to:

My father Amédée, lucid and spry at 101 years old, thank you for your inspiration.
The 7 billion people on planet Earth, thank you all for being my teachers.
Brandy, my deep appreciation for your caring recommendation.
Dr. Bruce Lipton, thank you for your confidence in me.
Dr. Joel Wallach, thank you for your gracious foreword.
Venessa, thank you for your insight and motivation.
Alain, thank you for your encouragement and help.
Cousin John, thank you for your loyal devotion.
Melinda, thank you for your extraordinary care.
Herbert, thank you for your editorial support.
Peter Stewart, thank you for your impetus.
My appreciators, thank you for choosing me.
My detractors, thank you for your boost.
My following, thank you for your trust.

FOREWORD

Therapist Sri Regine Lherisson-Bey has put together a broad collection of toxic forms of pollution to look at in relation to their effects on health, obesity, and excessive body weight.

This collection of data on health and toxicity as it relates to pollution has been grouped together in her book *How to Detoxify Your Life Naturally*.

Therapist Lherisson-Bey quite accurately looks at human disease from two aspects – nutrition and toxicity. Malnutrition produces the 'munchies', 'snacking', and 'cravings' which then put the malnourished individual in a position of being at higher risk of consuming toxic substances.

The book is practical from the standpoint that it educates the beginner as well as the expert on options regarding how to protect and repair the Earth, humans, and even animals.

Humans and the Earth must be free of pollution if we are going to be free of diseases.

Dr. Joel D. Wallach, B.S., D.V.M., N.D.
Author of the bestselling book
Dead Doctors Don't Lie

Biography

Dr. Joel Wallach is a recipient of the 2011 Klaus Schwarz Award recognizing the work of pioneers in the field of trace element research. A biomedical research pioneer, Joel D. Wallach, DVM, ND spent more than 40 years in the field of Veterinary Medicine, observing and researching the effects of individual nutrients on animal health, before becoming a Naturopathic Physician in 1982. Today, Dr. Wallach is renowned for his groundbreaking research on the health benefits of selenium and other minerals. He currently dedicates his time to lecturing throughout the world on the therapeutic benefits of vitamins and minerals, and on lobbying the U.S. Food and Drug Administration on behalf of the dietary supplement industry.

Dr. Wallach obtained a Bachelor of Science in Agriculture from the University of Missouri in 1962, with a major in Animal Husbandry (Nutrition) and a minor in Field Crops and Soils. In 1964, he was awarded a Doctorate in Veterinary Medicine (DVM), also from the University of Missouri. Thereafter, Dr. Wallach completed a three-year (1965-68) post-doctoral fellowship at The Center for the Biology of Natural Systems at Washington University in St. Louis, Missouri. In 1982, he obtained a Doctorate in Naturopathic Medicine (ND) from the National College of Naturopathic Medicine in Portland, Oregon.

Introduction

Our world has become very toxic. It is a known fact that toxicity contributes to ill health, obesity, and excessive body weight. The World Watch Institute has just reported that worldwide, nearly two billion people are overweight and obese. This count represents a 25% increase over the statistics of the year 2002. The number of overweight and obese people in the ten poorest countries in the world is at 18% while the number of overweight and obese people in the ten richest countries has been estimated at 70%. The situation is now considered epidemic since the numbers continue to increase. In spite of countless diets, pills, gyms, surgical procedures, books, recordings, television shows, Internet sites, etc., massively used to address the issue, the number of afflicted people seems to be growing. Most issues with excess body fat and other health problems are related to the toxicity of our food supply and the nutritionally deficient foods that the supply contains. This problem affects men and women, children and adults alike.

In January 2013, Dr. Otis Brawley, chief medical officer for the American Medical Association reported in an interview with CNN News: " The obesity epidemic is also affecting cancer rates in a very negative way. Indeed, obesity is the second leading cause of cancer. More than a dozen cancers -- from breast and prostate cancer to pancreatic and colon cancer -- have been linked to America's epidemic of high caloric intake and lack of physical activity. While 15% of adults were obese in 1970, more than 35% were obese in 2010. Even more concerning, 4% of children aged 6 to 11 were obese in 1970; 20% of that group were obese in 2010. While overall there is a significant decline in cancer mortality, the obesity epidemic is continuing to push the cancer mortality rate upward."

The bulk of our population is still mostly unaware of the connection between high toxicity and disease. Our food supply contains more than 10,000 chemical toxins and barely 300 of them have been tested for safety. Although toxicity affects everyone, people with excess body fat are more likely to store toxins that are hard to release. Scientists have recently reported that the toxicity problem is so crucial, young people are dying of toxicity-related illnesses at a higher rate than ever recorded in history. This means that the parents of this century are more likely to bury their children rather than the children burying them, a situation that translates into a historically unprecedented phenomenon.

It is becoming more obvious now that the obesity and weight issues are caused by different factors, mostly environmental toxicity and malnutrition involving overfeeding with food products that have little to no nutritional value. Usually, food products of this type are also toxic. When malnourished, eventually, the body in its search for better nutrition experiences insatiable hunger that foodstuff low in nutrients but high in toxins can never satisfy the body from hunger.

For any type of problem relating to toxicity, solutions do exist, at least for the most part. However, solutions involve a combination of workable processes that must be utilized in synchronicity. While most people are looking at only one or two processes in search of sensible solutions, it is essential to address the issue thoroughly and quickly by initiating change. Now that we understand that most of what has been done to help the ill-ness issue does not work too well, only an action-oriented paradigm shift can activate the effectiveness of the solutions we explore.

> *"The significant problems we have cannot be solved at the same level of thinking we were at when we created them."*
>
> ~ Albert Einstein

Bridging the gap

This book is a timely guide intended to bridge the gap between current weight control methodologies and the changing needs of the affected population of overweight and obese people. On their search for remedies, most people talk about 'taking' something or 'trying' a new pill, diet, gym program, liposuction, gastric bypass surgery, or shake. What seems to be grossly ignored by the average person however is the urgent need to change their lifestyle, learn to detoxify, learn to nourish oneself properly, and keep working on the changes for measurable results. It is puzzling to hear people talk about what they are 'taking' to 'lose weight', while they should consider what to 'change' or 'stop taking', or 'let go of' in order to 'release the extra weight' with consistency. What counts is not so much what we must take as much as what we are to stop taking and start replacing with healthier choices. The most overlooked fact in weight management is the understanding that toxins and malnutrition are major factors in the weight issue, and they are stressors operating multi-dimensionally within the body. Toxins and malnutrition affect both the body and the mind.

In various degrees, everyone on earth is toxic. Fat cells are toxic cells. Whether the toxicity resides in the body on the physical, emotional, or spiritual level, and usually on all levels, it has to be addressed multi-dimensionally for proper resolution. When people learn to shed their toxins, let go of their negative emotions, and embrace a healthier, non-toxic lifestyle, then constructive change starts occurring.

A lot of people are overfed, but because what they are feeding themselves with is not real food, but 'food stuff', they end up being malnourished and nutritionally deficient. Nowadays, some of the symptoms of malnourishment are: excess weight, obesity, poor muscle tone, mental dysfunction, and degenerative illnesses, just to name a few.

In America today, there is a high consumption of fast food, convenience food, junk food, and diet drinks. They mostly provide the body with a high level of processed sugar, saturated fats, fried high carbohydrates, and preservatives. Such foodstuff does not really nourish the body but robs from it by taking its existing nutrients for energetic compensation. Junk food with empty calories will steal from the body whatever amount of nutrients it contains and leave it devitalized, starving for more processed foods. When feeling assaulted or starved, the body receives triggers to prepare itself for combat and simply starts producing more... fat.

OBESITY RATE BY COUNTRY COMPARISON

Source: commons.wikimedia.org

This book is about bringing an innovative and durable solution to the weight issue by way of detoxification of one's life and person in the most complete sense of the term. After proper detoxification, the next step is to remedy malnutrition through replenishment. A lot of people do not know what to eat and how to eat. In both the detoxification and the replenishment phases, people are to upgrade their diet and engage in a regular exercise program.

Whether someone is looking to release excessive weight, control stress, or seeking to maintain a higher level of wholeness in their life, this manual has all it takes to create the quality awareness that many people are searching for. Our manual addresses the most major issues that are known to contribute to cellular toxicity in today's world. It explores practically all of the multiple avenues now being utilized in energy medicine for the purpose of attaining optimum wellness.

Dr. Mehmet Oz recently commented on the Oprah Winfrey Show: *"As we get a better understanding about how little we know about the body, we begin to realize that the next big frontier in medicine is energy medicine."* For all practical purposes, we have included in the book a whole inventory of modalities that are used by energy medicine practitioners and reported to be making positive differences in people's lives. We have covered all types of detoxification processes, that besides having withstood the test of time, have been proven safe and effective. The fact that all the modalities mentioned herein are non-toxic and life-enhancing, makes this material a safe and valuable guide for all sincere seekers of wellness. Any reader looking to make a difference in their health, their attitudes, and their quality of life in general has found a treasure in this book.

This material also assists in making the connection between environmental pollution and bodily pollution which leads to disease and fatalities. The understanding of the connection will help raise consciousness on how people can endeavor to be less mindlessly destructive toward Earth and therefore themselves, and be more motivated to reduce their carbon footprint.

The information we present

The information presented herein is a very comprehensive and thorough summary of a vast body of knowledge that can serve anyone who is at integrity with their search for solutions. Many aspects of the full detoxification process may at times be either neglected or ignored by even some competent and conscientious health practitioners. Such aspects may appear to be irrelevant or unimportant to them, and in some cases, be even unknown. For the sake of good conscience and wholeness, basically all aspects of the detoxification process are covered in this manual as an effort to create useful awareness; it is the multitude of overlooked data that can sometimes help discover what works and what does not. This works best when pertinent data is scrutinized, assembled, and properly utilized.

Psychophysiology, the science of the mind-body connection, shows ample evidence that self-detoxification works well when it comes to improving health. It works best when a follow-up involves complete rebalancing through proper nutrition, adequate hydration, and attitudinal healing. These are the most logical and workable steps in any natural weight management process.

Whole-brain solutions vs. left brain solutions

The purpose of this book is to create awareness on whole-brain solutions for all types of toxicity issues. Those who seek will find the solutions and can utilize them for relief. This book does not purport to be a scientific or medical manual.

The value of levity

At the end of each chapter in this book, there is space allotted for levity. Not only is laughter considered to be potent medicine, but also it is known to help us connect more effectively with our self while experiencing some commonality with our fellow humans. For inspiration, we can follow the example of Dr. Norman Cousins, who was a chiropractor and one of the people who were most aware of the mind-body connection in his time. After being diagnosed with a terminal illness, he was able to turn his life around and heal himself by choosing to incorporate joyfulness and laughter in his daily life. Norman Cousins was portrayed in 1984 in a television movie entitled: Anatomy of an Illness, based on his book: *Anatomy of an Illness as Perceived by the Patient: Reflections on Healing*. Dr. Cousins, an Adjunct Professor of Medical Humanities for the School of Medicine at the University of California, Los Angeles, conducted research on the biochemistry of human emotions. He discovered that the key to fighting illness was to maintain a positive attitude. After he was diagnosed with heart disease, he chose to heal himself by using laughter and Vitamin C. He managed to live thirty-six years after the diagnosis.

As Dr. Cousins has inspired the world to do with his joyfulness-based self-healing process, we can choose to experience a higher level of joy daily by utilizing levity and acknowledging the power of our mind to heal. Laughter causes our body to detoxify and also release beneficial hormones called endorphins. Many health professionals have come to label laughter: "The best medicine." Scientific American Magazine has corroborated this fact, as seen in the following link: http://www.scientificamerican.com/article.cfm?id=why-laughter-may-be-the-best-pain-medicine.

Very much like Norman Cousins, E. E. Cummings has also inspired the world by saying: "The most wasted of all days is one without laughter.". Because laughter clears our energy systems, promotes optimism and even relieves bodily pain, we can remember that it is vital to use humor daily on one's journey to self-detoxification.

Humor is detoxifying in the sense that it clears our energy systems from emotional burdens. It relaxes our muscles, upgrades our oxygen levels, and increases our neuropeptides count. All of this contributes to reinforcing our immune system therefore affording us more powerful cellular immunity. Since we learn best when we are relaxed, and since humor puts us in better dispositions, the reader will find value in the levity.

You can often tell how toxic or non-toxic someone is either by how uptight they are or how responsive they are to levity. Joy is such an important factor in healing and recovery that, every time we have the opportunity to incorporate it in our daily life, we are to consider it a healing opportunity to use, propagate, and be grateful for.

In an article entitled Humor and Health, Paul E. McGhee, Ph.D., a developmental psychologist and author of fifty scientific articles and thirteen books on humor elaborates on the matter of self-healing through optimism as follows:

> *"Whether or not you get sick depends on your body's ability to fight off infection and disease. In 1980 (prior to the discovery of the AIDS virus), the departing editor of the New England Journal of Medicine, Dr. Franz Ingelfinger, estimated that 85% of all human illnesses are curable by the body's own healing system. We now know that building a positive focus in your life plays an important role in supporting the body's ability to do this.*
>
> *The body's healing system responds favorably to positive attitudes, thoughts, moods, and emotions (e.g., to love, hope, optimism, caring, intimacy, joy, laughter, and humor), and negatively to negative ones (hatred, hopelessness, pessimism, indifference, anxiety, depression, loneliness, etc.). So you want to organize your life to maintain as positive a focus as possible."*

A functional way to upgrade our vibrational frequency is to utilize humor in our daily conversations or just for our self-enjoyment. Because humor – that is, clean humor, of course – cleanses our system by raising our frequency, it is to be an integral part of any healing regimen.

This book presents solutions-based awareness in the best interest of the people. Even though it is an eye opener on many hazards that affect all on Earth, – and the Earth itself – it uses an encouraging tone to guide and empower people. It can serve both beginners who do not know where to start when it comes to detoxification as well as advanced practitioners of self-detoxification. When adults act with conscious awareness of facts, they can make informed choices. Democracy presupposes an informed citizenry. This book is all about information and choices: its wealth of data is suitable for all sincere seekers. Whether people are looking to know how to sensibly exercise their own choices and detoxify themselves on all levels while also detoxifying the environment, this book has the answers. May it serve you well!

<h1 style="text-align:center">Chapter 1</h1>

<h1 style="text-align:center">There Are No Isolated Structures</h1>

"When people go within and connect with themselves, they realize they are connected to the universe and they are connected to all living things."

~ Armand Dimele

Because most of the material in this book deals with the concept of detoxification of the self for the purpose of attaining wholeness on all levels, we will first cover the prerequisites of the understanding of wholeness. The word wholeness means completeness, fullness of harmony in its integrity. It also implies connectedness in purity and elevating ways. The construct of connectedness is huge and requires clarification of its general understanding.

We are one with a universal collective

It is important for us to be conscious of the fact that all of life's structures are inter-connected. Many people may find it incredulous that all beings and all things are energetically connected. At a subtle energetic level, every organism is connected to the collective of all organisms. There are people who, when they become aware of this fact, experience such a level of discomfort that they retreat into denial or avoidance. If our construct is that of separation and superiority over those we feel separated from, then discomfort and denial will be part of the reality check. The perceived separation or boundary is multifold and in general, is of a racial, geographical, political, financial, educational, or religious nature, among others. The separation was created over aeons of time – for an infinity of reasons – in order to build our societies. From a geopolitical point of view, tracking and managing society's individual members, serves to bring about the extreme complexity that is necessary for humans to experience an evolutionary process.

"If you wish to understand the Universe, think of energy, frequency and vibration."
~ Nikola Tesla

1

Albert Einstein has said:

Since no one can ever successfully alter the immutable laws of physics, a simple analysis of the interconnectedness of all things allows us to observe an infinity of subdivisions within the concept of connectedness.

Theorem of holistic knowledge:
Any subject is a composite
of all other subjects.

People function as individuals, with various degrees of autonomy and free will, physically detached from each other and also mentally detached from others by virtue of the existence of the construct referred to as the ego. The ego allows us to be conscious of our own individuality which is a form of compartmentalization. Regardless of the individuality, on some energetic level, all people and things are connected. The connectedness constitutes a message that it is through symbiotic interaction that survival and evolution can be successfully experienced. This success however also depends on how the connected individuals are able to fulfill the conditions of harmonious symbiosis. Humans usually feel safer when knowing that they are part of a bigger structure, a whole unit, whether it is their community or the universe itself.

Problems with the collective

Living in a collective is never fully harmonious unless the collective has individual units that are themselves harmonious. Each individual unit carries its own sense of individuality and own signature frequency, a lot of it is pathological. The collective is, on some level more of a petri dish for the development of all categories of issues leading to either agreement, neutrality, or conflict. In many cases, it is mostly conflict. Depending on the level of development of the individual souls that are members of the collective, individual ego creates all sorts of reasons for initiating conflict. More often than not, the conflicts are artificial or contrived. In all cases they serve as part of the learning experiences that humans are here to create for themselves. In this school called life, even conflict is a parameter used to assess humans' ability to function within their community and their willingness to evolve as a specie.

This situation regarding the survival of the collective has brought the necessity of initiating methods that serve to feed the collective quickly and abundantly. Based on reported history, in the beginning of this civilization's cycle, most of the daily preoccupations were with agriculture, farming, fishing, and animal husbandry which allowed people to trade and barter in ways that kept them focused on raising their family in nurturing and protective ways, have a social connection, take time to love, focus on the arts and cultural endeavors. This had allowed the people in the collective to be fed in nourishing and sustainable ways that also honored the environment. With the advent of the industrial revolution, the daily preoccupations of the collective became modified. The lifestyle of the collective switched from manual labor to machinery, technological manipulation, and the artificial handling of all aspects of life, from feeding methods to self-entertainment. Many people flocked to large cities, creating major urban agglomerations that came with out-of-control pollution of the air, water, soil, and everything else. The agglomerations also came with lower quality food and water, excessive production of artificial waste that is not always recycled or recyclable; soon after a preoccupation with artificial goods began to prevail. A lot of such artificial goods have contributed to desecrating the environment, all in the name of progress. The new way of living has been focused on high technology, machinery, speed of production, most of which entailed overwhelming production of plastics. Even entertainment leads to the overproduction of plastic material for audio and videographic purposes. With this new lifestyle, the social connection became confused. For many people, love turned to fear, nurture turned to exploitation and predatory practices; even for the very young and the very old, social and sexual perversions became mainstream, the rate of mental and physical illnesses soared. This stemmed from a pronounced disconnection from nature. The life cycle of the collective has become disturbed to the point that people no longer know how to eat, when to eat, what to eat, what is real food and what is not, when to sleep, when to work and when to play. Even though the evolution of the collective into a more mechanical, more robotic, quasi- automatic creation looks more organized and more controllable, it also relates to more people being electronically connected, entertained, a situation that leads to less interactive connections therefore more neuroses, a less human-like sense of fulfillment, and consequently, more toxicity. As the planet was being transformed into a testing ground for toxicity, all sorts of industries sprung up. Many of them have had a covert agenda to profit from the people by encouraging ignorance, greed, and a contrived sense of powerlessness. They have been promoting toxicity under the guise of providing entertainment or social services to the masses.

Subdivisions within the connectedness of the collective

We are either fully conscious or somewhat aware of our connectedness with all things; we also know that within the whole, there are numerous subdivisions; there are many reasons for the necessity of creating subdivisions and there are infinite implications regarding the structure of the subdivisions. The subdivisions have been established for an organizational purpose. Even though they have some connotation with separation, they still contain the same program of connectedness within their structure. Within subdivisions, all beings are still connected to one another, in one way or another. It is this interconnectedness which eventually allows us to understand the sophistication of the relationship between the one and the many in proportion to oneness as opposed to division. The globe is divided into continents that contain subcontinents. Continents contain clusters of countries, such as the Eastern Block, for instance. Within countries and societies, there is the division of social classes or strata. Within the classes or strata, there are subclasses of people. The subclasses usually involve communities, sub-communities, groups, special interest groups, gangs, mobs, federations, fraternities, associations, tribes, down to the traditional family structure. Within each of the mentioned substructures, there is division. Even in families some people choose to express more love for certain members than for others. Besides being indicative of a lack mentality, this behavior denotes a moral conflict within the self, and self- conflicted people are toxic.

Societal structures

Each society has its own divisions and subdivisions. Their criteria usually overlap and all societies share similarities. The most enduring concept of social classes is its subdivision into strata. In all cultures, society is structured as: the upper class, the middle class, and the lower class. A lot of our society's agenda is not often graspable at least regarding the concept of long-range agenda. Many societal constructs contribute to collective and individual toxicity.

SOCIETY'S COVERT STRUCTURE

Categories	Characteristics	Standards		Agenda
The upper class	. The ruling class . The investing class . The entrepreneurial class . The intellectual class	Benevolent/Adjusted subtype	We think for you We speak for you We educate you We create the infrastructure We like order and aesthetics We eat organic gourmet food	We control you We watch you We distract you
		Criminal/Maladjusted subtype	We think for you We take from you We live off your labor We deceive you We enslave you We create biotech food for you We steal from you through adhesion contracts We institutionalize you We slaughter you with impunity We decide for you We mis-educate you We keep you sick We eat biotech gourmet food	We promote imperialistic supremacy through elite education We create toxins We sell you toxins We convince you that toxins are good for you
The middle class	. The working class . The entrepreneurial subclass . The investing subclass . The intellectual subclass	Benevolent/Adjusted subtype	We think for ourselves if it is safe We assimilate you We educate our children We show you the way We work for them / ourselves We study you We eat everything	We follow each other We keep up with the Joneses We follow the leader
		Criminal / Maladjusted subtype	We want what you have We take and steal from you We mis-educate you We institutionalize you We murder you then we get prosecuted We eat anything, especially fast and junky	We watch sports and celebrities on TV We want to be like them We buy / sell toxins
The lower class	. The working subclass . The manual laborer class . The slave class . The public charge class	Benevolent / Adjusted subtype	We work for you We grow your food We count on you We eat everything	We do as you say We follow you
		Criminal / Maladjusted subtype	We live off you We con you into feeding us We mug you We kill you then we get executed We trash the infrastructure We speak trash / we play trash music We eat anything, especially fast, junky, and even scraps	We obey you We watch you on TV We promote anti-education We consume toxins

Conflict within the self translates into conflict with others

Within the collective and all aspects of the subdivisions, including the nuclear family, if one unit is not at peace with itself, inevitably, it will engage in conflict with the other units. From sibling rivalry to warfare between one nation and another, conflict affects all entities in all strata of the societal structure. Most of the problems begin when one unit or one group starts asserting its superiority or authority over the other for ego gratification or mercenary gain. Usually authority is greatly abused by units who do not know how to handle power. It is rare to find anyone gifted with enough wisdom to handle power benevolently, equitably, and gracefully, all the time. In all cases, anyone expressing conflict or dis-harmony is affected by one constant: personal toxicity.

When we take a good look at the laws of physics, it brings up the realization that our thoughts and words create our reality. This is a fact that is rather painful for certain humans to admit. The caveat that we create our reality forces us humans to face that we are then responsible for our own life's conditions; such conditions include physical wellness or illness. It takes courage to face the hurt one has caused to the self and others, particularly if one has been trained to assign responsibility to authority figures. In a world ruled by authority figures demanding blind obedience, it is the most compliant people whose gullibility is the most easily exploited.

With over seven billion people living on planet Earth, the world is a huge project to manage; divisions – natural, artificial, and virtual – have been created for the purpose of maintaining order within structures on our planet. Often, the construct of division is used, or more precisely misused, for the purpose of perpetrating evil. It is not so much the division itself that is a problem as much as the misguided attitudes toward the division. When organizational division is used to malign others then it is a big problem for the collective. This can be seen in all levels of the structure. That is why over several millennia, the earth's population has seen a whole range of conflicts based on the intolerance of one group toward the other. The conflicts have been mostly in this order: from personal, political, familial, tribal, racial, religious, financial, intellectual, sexual, to intergalactic. For instance, when one special interest group endeavors to malign another because they are uncomfortable about the other group's differences, that entails inevitable conflict. For certain people, groups, or organizations, differences equate threat. Even though certain individuals may not be stepping on others' toes, if they are perceived as different – therefore as a threat -- then they are treated as if they are 'bad' – not different, just 'bad'. In other cases, some individuals may be perpetrating acts that are downright immoral, even amoral, but yet, are tolerated because their actions serve a political agenda. Most of the time, the agenda serves the enrichment of those from the group of people that considers themselves as possessing superior knowledge, more power, or both. In just about every case where abuse of power is involved, the abuse is related to a misplaced or sick ego. Wherever there is misplaced or sick ego, there is likely an issue with mismanaged emotions and uncontrolled toxicity. Usually, toxicity affecting the emotional body is at the root of just about every conflict, whose levels may range from personal to intergalactic. Toxic emotions are the opposite of personal serenity. When we are toxic, our thought processes are tainted with negativity. This negativity eventually spreads from one person to another and contaminates the whole structure like a virus. Fear serves to maintain duality and overall, duality perpetuates toxicity.

Emma Restall Orr offers a clear explanation of the dichotomy pertaining to the issue of connectedness and separation: *"The important element is the way in which all things are connected. Every thought and action sends shivers of energy into the world around us, which affects all creation. Perceiving the world as a web of connectedness helps us to overcome the feelings of separation that hold us back and cloud our vision. This connection with all life increases our sense of responsibility for every move, every attitude, allowing us to see clearly that each soul does indeed make a difference to the whole."*

The Internet is one of the greatest examples of how everything is interconnected; it is in fact, a symbol of how we are transcending connectivity limitations as we continue to evolve. In our evolutionary process, we as beings with infinite capabilities, are resonating with each other through thought frequencies and feelings.

One unit contaminates the whole

In general, the fear of one can be transmitted to others. Because connecting is part of our experience on planet Earth, connectedness, as all things, also comes with its own set of problems. One serious issue with connectedness is that of energetic contamination. Wherever there is contact, there is a risk of contamination. People are on different levels of frequencies depending on what their lifestyle is and what kind of thoughts they are processing. Because we are all connected to all things, we also incur the risk of contaminating one another. Being part of the solution is more elevating than being part of the problem; we must focus on solutions because, if humans can contaminate each other, they can also de-contaminate each other. This book offers sensible solutions for self-detoxification and also the detoxification and decontamination of affected people for the purpose of healing our selves and humanity.

People's states of being run the whole gamut of emotions, from absolute rage to inspirational serenity. Most people do not stay consistently at one particular set point regarding their emotions. The fluctuations in people's emotions depend on individual maturity leading to their ability to handle those emotions. In general, purity of mind and body contributes to a higher level of emotional strength in certain individuals. People with a higher level of toxicity than average humans contribute to infecting the environment that the less toxic people live in. This toxicity usually manifests itself in the form of artificial conflicts that toxic individuals engineer. They have a knack for creating conflict in their own lives and also the lives of those around them.

Some beings abhor conflict whereas some others thrive on it. It is a sad fact that in our society today, conflict is used and overused for entertainment. Many people are addicted to the display of toxic material that over-emphasizes conflict. This is a situation that has to do with different ranges of thought frequencies that coexist but are more attuned to discordant energies. Someone must be already toxic to express enjoyment for discordant energies that clash with one another because they are the antithesis of peace. When someone is toxic, most of the time, they are not at peace. Regardless of who is around them, they will find a reason to express impatience, attack someone, eventually get into screaming fits, insults, challenging, blaming, and condemning. Even when there is no reason for conflict they will create one; by a self-righteous feat of the ego, such people will surely find a way to give their conflict an accent of legitimacy. Once hey feel that their attack is justified, their ego is content. There exists some people that no amount of logical reasoning can bring to reason. *You can lead a fool to wisdom but you can't make him think.*

It can be enlightening to observe how some individuals may be exposed to wisdom over and over again, and yet, never understand the need to align with it. Every person on earth possesses a modicum of wisdom, in various degrees, and everyone has their own point of view. Points of views also come with blind sides that just about everyone has to some degree. It is when different views are properly evaluated and measured that a sensible opinion can be formed. Many people are looking at issues in ways that can be considered to equate exploring one side of an elephant, as an analogy. Some may look just at one side and conclude that this is the way the whole elephant is. They are taking the long route to their evolution but that is a choice.

> *"No great improvements in the lot of mankind are possible until a great change takes place in their mode of thought."*
> ~ John Stuart Mill

Our Earth contains people of all types, convictions, attitudes, mental states, and agendas. They range from the most benevolent humanitarians, philanthropists, and visionaries to the most vile criminals, lowly thieves, imposters, liars, deceivers, and deranged derelicts.

Due to the very large number of people living on the planet, it is not possible to have homogeneity of character or behavior in the collective. It is the extreme differences that exist in the human collective that constitutes the material for learning how to reconcile opposites. As seen above, some people revel in conflict and others live in serenity: the difference resides in the different ranges of frequencies they operate by. People come together or stay apart, depending on what level of vibrational frequency they are resonating with at any point in time.

Woodrow Wilson has allegedly said: *"If a dog will not come to you after having looked you in the face, you should go home and examine your conscience."* One of the main issues in our world is the lack of self-examination. Many people are on automatic pilot and would not even think of examining their conscience. They are programmed to not even think for themselves on some level, and that program entails shifting blame onto others to defend their ego. Blame shifting indicates irresponsibility and when we have to deal with a large number of irresponsible people, then it is a huge problem. Take a look at the issues society has with drunk driving, texting while operating public and private vehicles, child sexual abuse, human trafficking, etc., and these are just a few examples of what irresponsibility is. In his Apology, Plato wrote: *"An unexamined life is not worth living."* When one learns to examine their own life, their vibrational frequency also rises. If one's personal frequency is low, one is toxic.

Everything is about frequencies. We humans are sophisticated bio-resonant machines with our mind constantly impacting our body, and on one or more subtle levels, the minds of others. In order for people of higher frequencies to survive around those of the lower frequencies, there are certain requirements that must be fulfilled. First one must be mentally balanced. Second, one must decide what aspect of the world to deal with. We can choose to live in a world of peace or a toxic world of strife. For us to accomplish such a goal, we must purify our thoughts and feelings in order to remain within the normal range of a higher level of frequency.

We often see people argue for their limiting views of the human connectedness and say that since we are physically separate, then there is no connectedness. This statement often occurs, especially in circles where some people are ethnically different from others. Among billions of worldviews, this is only one pertaining to the presumed lack of connectedness. If we are what we breathe, what we drink, and what we eat; and if we are breathing the same air as everybody else is breathing; if we are drinking the water that we all use for growing food, preparing our meals, taking showers, brush our teeth, expectorate, and flush our waste, aren't we all sharing energetic frequencies and vibrating like one as a collective?

Being one is one thing, and being unified and harmonious is another. When even one unit is toxic, then the whole collective also contains the frequency of toxicity. Detoxification of the units, one at a time, can help the collective evolve at a higher level of harmony and wholeness. Because we live in a world of duality, functioning on Earth entails having to coexist with units exhibiting different levels of toxicity.   Even though it may never be possible to decontaminate the sum total of the collective, any effort toward self detoxification can contribute to collective detoxification, and can eventually alleviate the toxic condition on some level. If the improvement ever reaches critical mass, then the frequency of the collective will have greatly improved also.

A lack of structural connectedness contributes to an unhealthy lifestyle

Many people complain that dieting has not helped them solve the problem of excessive body fat afflicting them. They do not understand how to improve their situation but could solve their problem within one day if they were only willing to listen and learn how certain structures operate. In many cases, people perish due to a lack of knowledge. When one is capable of understanding the role of the connectedness of all structures, then the toxicity issue starts finding resolution. The same resolution applies to excessive weight and related health problems too.

The average overweight person lives a lifestyle that makes them a toxic time bomb,. The following scenario will be used as an example to describe the dynamics of that kind of lifestyle and show where it is faulty. The subject, Toxic Time Bomb, hereafter referred to as TTB:

- Gets up but does not take the time to connect to source energy and express gratitude for being alive another day. (Disconnection from source.)
- May not always create the time to connect with the family members of the household for a gesture of affection or kindness. (Disconnection from the energy of love.)
- Gets ready for work by taking a shower with chlorinated tap water introducing multiple chemicals in the body through the pores; washes their hair with shampoo containing sodium lauryl sulfate; conditions their hair with products laced with parabens; puts on a generous amount of deodorant loaded with aluminum, parabens and other toxic chemicals;
- Saturates their skin with lotion containing propylene glycol, after using shampoo laced with sodium lauryl sulfate; (Disconnection from environmental awareness.)
- Avoids breakfast at all costs. Rushing to the appointment is a priority. (Disconnection from self- nurture.)

- Stops by a fast food place to buy pesticides-laden coffee prepared with tap water, poured into a styrofoam cup covered with a phthalates-emitting plastic lid. (Disconnection from home; ignorance of environmental protection and non-toxic self-care.)
- Gets to their appointment or work until mid-day, therefore skipping breakfast. The Toxic Time Bomb is now hungry, dizzy, irritable, and their blood sugar level is out of whack. (Disconnection from nurture, self-love and self-respect.)
- Grabs a fast food sandwich made of genetically modified organisms (GMO) and eats it on the run by mid-day. (Disconnection from serenity and self-nurture.)
- Buys a large package of TV dinner – more fast food. (Disconnection from nurture.)
- Buys and carries a large package of bottled water – more phthalates and Bisphenol-A, and also more acidifying material for the body. This contributes to more plastic that ends up littering the environment. (Disconnection from nurture and environmental care.)
- Rushes on the highway to get home just on time to catch the news or nightly TV program contributing to negative programming, prolonged exposure to electromagnetic frequencies and deceptive subliminal messages (Disconnection from wholeness.)
- Gets home, microwaves the TV dinner and consumes it quickly while watching endless TV programming convincing them to buy more TV dinners and more bottled water. Now there is more plastic packaging that has accumulated and is likely to be thrown away rather than being recycled. Instead of taking a walk after dinner to promote digestion and curb obesity, the TTB lies on the couch for hours to relax while being programmed by default and producing excess weight. (Disconnection from true nurture and environmental concern.)
- Lies on the couch for the next few hours to watch extended TV programming contributing to pineal gland damage. (Disconnection from the self and others.)
- Falls asleep on the couch soon after the heavy meal while the food rots in the stomach promoting an overweight condition and obesity (Self neglect.)
- Wakes up groggy to use dental hygiene products containing toxic petrochemicals that are known endocrine disruptors (Unconscious self-abuse.)
- Goes to bed, spends the rest of the might tossing, gets up at times to self-medicate and wondering why they suffer from a sleep disorder. (Disconnection from self-knowledge)

It is a bewildering fact that many toxic time bombs spend most, if not all, of their spare time on a couch watching TV. A more wholesome activity could be walking in a park or a mall, or engaging in mind- enhancing social interaction. The same people who harbor such lifestyle usually complain of decreased energy levels and poor muscle tone. A sedentary lifestyle is said to contribute to obesity and cancer besides other ills. A walk in a park can help increase oxygen intake that usually revitalizes the body. A low oxygen count brought on by a sedentary lifestyle is a factor that contributes to degenerative illnesses. Excessive TV viewing is sometimes a covert way to initiate ongoing distraction and avoid being in touch with the self or interacting with others. Because TV viewing is neither interactive nor conversational, prolonged exposure to it deactivates a part of the mind and eventually contributes to dullness of the senses. On the other hand, there are covert subliminal messages in advertising that are undetectable to TV viewers. Covert subliminal messages encoded in advertisements can be dishonest, unethical, and deceptive enough to trick a viewer into desiring to buy products they do not need or are not in their best interest. A lot of the time, these products are sold under the guise of affording more free time to the viewer but end up making their life and the environment more toxic. When people have more free time, they often spend it in front of their TV anyway; this situation eventually causes them to be more programmed and desire to buy more... products.

People who are toxic time bombs could make healthier choices such as: connecting with loved ones for better emotional health, filter the water in their shower to prevent the absorption of harmful chemicals. Such chemicals are known to cause brain fog and multiple other symptoms; some people could benefit from choosing to get up 20 minutes earlier to prepare their breakfast, the most important meal of the day. It takes the same amount of time, or less, to prepare organic coffee with filtered water at home than it takes to drive to a fast food place and wait in line to buy it. Another advantage people would get from making her own coffee is that there is no extra packaging to throw away; one can choose to eat nurturing, nutritious food instead of consuming genetically modified foodstuff; one can also choose to eat a light dinner and later take a walk for better digestion and blood circulation. Industrial food not only is hazardous to health but it also contributes to environmental pollution.

When people of the earth fail to see their individual responsibility to be vanguards of the planet, then the environmental mess worsens due to a lack of accountability. With the overwhelming production and distribution of packaged water and packaged foodstuff – among countless other packaged products – people are not focusing on reusing and recycling. The people of ancient indigenous cultures lived with great reverence for the planet, protecting it from excessive waste by reusing and properly recycling their daily essentials. Systematic trashing of the planet with un-recyclable waste contaminates the soil, water, and air, therefore our food supply.

Eventually the pollution causes people to be diseased, unhappy, and dysfunctional. It is the very dysfunction that also brings about even more irresponsibility in the way the planet is treated. So the whole process is a catch 22. It is high time we wake up from this terrible apathy and start taking responsibility by making all aspects of our lives eco-friendly by adopting a greener, healthier, and non-toxic lifestyle.

For levity:

"You can live to be a hundred if you give up all the things that make you want to be a hundred."

~ Woody Allen

<h1 style="text-align:center">Chapter 2</h1>

<h1 style="text-align:center">Detoxification Begins at Home: Our Body</h1>

"The body is not a permanent dwelling, but a sort of inn which is to be left behind when one perceives that one is a burden to the host."

~ Seneca

Before the 1940s, in most countries, the majority of babies were born at home. In many countries around the world, a doctor or midwife would go to the home of a woman in labor and assist with the birth-giving process. Modern life has changed this lifestyle in various parts of the world; nowadays, particularly in so-called industrialized countries, most births occur in hospitals; a smaller number of births takes place in birthing centers. Our primary home is our body. Our mother's womb was our first home before we were born. Our brick-and-mortar dwelling is another home that is a symbol of the energetic human body housing the mind, spirit, and soul.

Our body is our true home

In reality, because we are spiritual beings having a human experience, and because our body is our true home, then we are always home. The body is a home that incubated within a home known as our mother's womb; we eventually grew up within an architectural structure which is our house; our house is a dwelling for our physical body until we are laid to rest in the ultimate home which is our Earth, that is within another home which is the macrocosm. This cycle goes to infinity and confirms that toxicity goes in cycles. If the earth is toxic, then our body becomes toxic and our offspring also becomes toxic. After conception, we incubate inside our mother's body; then after birth, we learn to adapt to an earthly life within our brick-and-mortar home or wherever we are raised. If the brick-and-mortar home is toxic, then we are likely to experience health issues that are known to affect people living in toxic homes. When our physical homes are toxic, our bodies become toxic.

As of the past few years, more and more toxins have been reported to accumulate in humans, even babies. Research studies are indicating that people's tissues are registering residues of plastic byproducts and traces of hazardous chemicals in an unprecedented way. This indicates the gravity of the situation because scientists have found hazardous chemicals to cause genetic mutations. Hazardous chemicals are in the air, the water, the food, and everything around us. It is in human's best interest to detoxify if they want to conceive properly and maintain a healthy progeny. For people who do not understand the repercussions of plastic overuse -- for their body and the environment -- it is essential to read this book's chapter on environmental toxicity.

The physical body is a reflection of the environment. Just as the earth has an ecosystem, the physical body has its own ecosystem. An ecosystem is home to an enormous number of organisms some of which are good and some of which are bad. Some of them are there to preserve life and others are there to kill. They are part of the cycle of life and death, just as it is for humans on the planet. If it were not for bad bacteria and mold, we would virtually have eternal life. For instance, the intestinal flora is composed of friendly bacteria that are part of the gastrointestinal system. When there is imbalance in the intestinal flora, the immune system experiences issues. The acid mantle is part of the eco-system of the skin which is part of the integumentary system. When there is imbalance in any of the bodily systems, then the whole body's structure ends up being compromised in various ways. The same way a house divided cannot stand, if the body is not whole, then it is compromised. It is imperative to take care of the body in ways that honor the spirit within to ensure its wholeness therefore its structural integrity.

We only live a harmonious life when our body's different systems are aligned with purity. Because nowadays for the most part, purity is a thing we have to work hard to obtain, it is important to detoxify and maintain the body as well as the brick-and-mortar home.

For levity:

"Home nowadays is a place where part of the family waits til the rest of the family brings the car back."

~ Earl Wilson

Chapter 3

Personal Space, Lifestyle, and Individual Toxicity

"We can have technology, prosperity, nice homes, and cars,
but at the same time, we must be conscious of what we are dumping into the water, the air, and our food."

~ Kevin Richardson

Quite often, one can tell at a glance, just looking at the outside of a home what the dweller's state of mind is, based on the appearance of the place. Because states of mind differ from one dweller to another, the types of dwelling also differ, each being a telltale sign of who is in, to a certain extent. The different types of mind states for house dwellers are categorized below. What follows will help you find out how you function in your personal space, based on your state of mind and level of consciousness that are also related to personal levels of toxicity. Money is not always a good yardstick for the type of space someone occupies and how toxic the space can be. Unless blatantly unacceptable, it does not matter much where the dwelling is and what type it is, what counts is its soundness and functionality. Some people live in immaculate studio apartments in modest communities while others live in filthy mansions in ostentatious neighborhoods. In general, the characteristics of the space where people live is an indication of the emotions such people are processing.

Different types of personal space

Type A: Pleasant, clean, orderly, comfortable, and welcoming.
Type B: Cluttered, somewhat organized, and uncomfortable.
Type C: Very cluttered, disorderly, filthy, disorganized, repulsive, and hazardous.

Different types of dwellers

1.   Dweller with an adjusted concept of personal space

<u>Personal traits:</u>

Dwellers of this type of space may be more adjusted physically and perhaps also mentally, due to healthier environmental conditions; they may enjoy a healthier lifestyle due to better nutrition, exercises, and a more sensible balance between work and play. Usually, people who manage to reach a good balance between their physical and financial life have more peace of mind and are more adjusted or happy. This does not mean that all wealthy people are more adjusted however. More adjusted dwellers are, to a certain extent, less toxic than people who are not as well adjusted. It is so mostly because of a similar sense of lifestyle passed down genetically, or because of their own determination to be well adjusted. These people may go through life with a harmonious state of being. Their living quarters usually express this state of being, reflecting sophistication, high aesthetics, and refinement in functionality. There often is meaning to the items that are part of the place's atmosphere. There seems to be a focus on intention. It does not matter much where the dwelling is and what type it is, what counts is its   soundness and functionality. This type of dweller is likely to create a palatial space out of any type of building, provided that it is in a harmonious environment. The characteristics of the living space of more adjusted people are usually an indication of the emotions they process. Their living space is clean, sweet smelling, well lit, harmoniously arranged, pleasantly decorated; fresh flowers may abound, and beautiful music resonates in the air. The dweller feels comfortable living there. Consequently, this type of person wants to nurture the self and loved ones with home-cooked foods; the dweller of such home is likely to ensure that they have an adequate supply of clean, potable drinking water, ample reserves of goods for times of inclement weather, or emergencies; this type of dweller also likes to surround themselves with beautiful plants and sounds. In a well adjusted dweller's home, the front and back yards are likely to have well-manicured lawns; usually, the home and yard have flowers and a pleasant landscape. The same holds true for the well-adjusted person's office, car, clothing and accessories; other indicators of adequate adjustment are: posture, work performance, speech, attitudes toward the self, other people, and pets. What is in such people's environment mirrors their state of mind. They are likely to seek health-oriented activities, and engage in meaningful, constructive conversations. This type of person prefers to live in pristine environments, near lakes, rivers, the ocean; they enjoy the great outdoors, and a lot of the time, away from the metropolis. People in this category are self-actualized members of society representing barely 3% of the population. This type of person is conscious and is most likely self-governed to a healthy extent.

<u>**Challenges:**</u>
This type of dweller may be rather solitary because they either work for themselves or live off their investment or they may be socially oriented. They may have a strong concept of personal boundaries and may even be considered to be of the isolationist kind if they are not a socialite.

Additionally, this type of dweller may suffer from obsessive-compulsive disorders, anxiety, inability to properly manage stress, issues related to eyesight due to excessive eye strain caused by excessive intellectual work, hernia, general debilitation, cardiovascular issues, excess weight gain, and bodily pains, especially if sedentary.

## 2.	Dweller with a divided concept of personal space

<u>**Personal traits:**</u>
This type of dweller is likely to live in a decent, well-kept space, and may have more than one or two homes. Money may not be an issue but unresolved childhood issues may be the cause of

serious blocks to personal development. This type of person might exhibit personality issues, featuring such traits as arrogance, mistrust, and low integrity. There may be a smile on their face or somewhat of an indication of self-assurance in their demeanor, but deep inside they may be unhappy, passive-aggressive people. They may work hard to afford to be well to do and live wherever they want, go wherever they want, but they may live in fear. They may appreciate the finer things in life and can afford to eat better than average people, so they may be in better physical shape than the rest of the population. This is a big plus mostly because they eat foods that keep them fit, and / or they exercise. They either work hard or work smart, or both. This type of dweller is rather semi-conscious. They may have a strong concept of personal boundaries but this construct is mostly due to fear of being exposed. This dweller is in quasi-actualization mode.

Challenges:

Because people in this category of dwellers are likely to be anally retentive, they are mostly constipated, uptight, and perhaps cynical. They may live in fear, which often translates into kidney disease and diabetes. Their living space, office, and car may be clean and orderly, but some of these people may be toxic and living in denial. They may be crude and contemptuous and have little regard for other people's feelings. They may feel dis-empowered on some personal level where they face challenges and maybe they are likely to have a tendency to whine. The feelings and needs of other people and humanity are not so much of their concern. They may be passive-aggressive and pay attention to hide their dysfunction rather well. After all, their image is important and face-saving is a priority. They seem to have a modicum of control over their external environment but their internal state is out of control. They may be extravagant, and extravagance can denote a narcissistic trait. They may pace the floor all night and let their perceived or real problems control their thinking day and night. They may swear loosely, even in the presence of children, because they may feel a sense of importance and invincibility due to their financial stability. Some of them may believe that they are exempt from civility or reverence. These people are likely to be irritable and intolerant of those around them. They may tolerate you, but it may be mostly because of the support you provide them, since as a matter of fact, they may not even like you. They are likely to mismanage their emotions and feel unable to handle guilt, shame, or grief. They may be self-indulgent and eccentric. All this may be an excuse for them to be addicted to overspending and / or recreational drugs. They may be compulsively crude or boastful about their achievements. They wish to be classy but lack the princely manners that go with class. They may be controlling due to greed and ego gratification.

3.   Dweller with a chaotic concept of personal space

Personal traits:

This is the construct of someone with a tormented mind. Because their mind is not at peace, he or she, the dweller of the space, is very much like a hurricane: unruly, disorderly, easily ticked off. Such people are likely to exhibit either schizophrenic or depressive traits accompanied by lethargy or apathy. When they get up, such people do not take the time to fix their bed: *messy bed equates messy head; messy head equates messy speech or behavior.* Chaotic dwellers leave a trail of disorder wherever they go in and around their place. This type of person is busy, very busy, always busy... most of the time, if not all of the time. This person also is likely to be the work-hard-play-hard type, of the most heavily entertained kind. With this type of person, even their entertainment is like work, and it usually is more toxic than necessary. Significant amounts of time are spent being mindlessly entertained in the name of relaxation. This type of person likes watching everything that goes on television: the news, every talk show, their favorite program, sports, gossips show, everything. They are busy being entertained, so they do not have the time, or the inclination, to clean after themselves. They leave their dishes piling up in the sink, their bills, beer bottles, and medication vials piling up near their couch, and these items may pile up for years. Since this type of dweller is likely to be on antidepressants, they also find that their energy level is low and their willpower virtually non-existent; they may leave their TV on all day and all night, even while they sleep. This habit adds insult to injury since TV transmitters emit electromagnetic frequencies and TV programming is encoded with toxic subliminal messages. In a chaotic dweller's home, drawers and cabinets are usually a mess, and the person spends an inordinate amount of time looking for anything they need. They often misplace their keys, telephone, gadgets, documents: an indication that they are not very present.

The dweller of a chaotic space may be edgy because of the frustrations and physiological fatigue that result from the lack of proper sleep. Due to unhappiness, they may not really care about themselves, their life, and others. Because of sleep-deprivation, they may be short-tempered and disrespectful. Also, because they do not like their environment and do not feel nurtured in it, they may look for shortcuts to cooking, cleaning, and going home. Such people may often take off to go outside and look for comfort food or drinks. These food items are usually highly acidic and include: coffee, fried foods, soft white bread, high carbohydrates, meats, and alcohol. When people stay long enough on this kind of diet, soon enough, hyper-acidosis takes over and they become arthritic, overweight, and obese. Overtime, they may exhibit fuzzy thinking, irritability, and road rage, besides memory loss and fast aging. This eventually augments unhappiness when these people must slow down and their quality of life is even worse than ever before. Once they are in pain often enough to seek medical assistance, they start taking other drugs on top of their anti- depressants. Then eventually, their physician most likely will have them undergo treatment for diabetes and or cancer to manage the symptoms that are now more pronounced.

In a chaotic space, the refrigerator is likely to be a biohazard, a potential time bomb that may contain old bread, green mold, black mold, and old rotten food. Mold spores can travel from one room to another and end up in the lungs through inhalation. Mold can also be responsible for a lot of recurrent respiratory issues and sinus infections. The chaotic space's kitchen sink and counter are likely to have black mold. Such place is also likely to have rodents and crawling pests.

A chaotic bathroom – just like the kitchen – is likely to have black mold and large amounts of dust. The dweller may say: *"What's the big deal if the place is moldy or dusty?"* Usually, this type of thinking indicates that it is the thinking itself that *is* the problem. In a neglected, toxic home, mold and dust are pervasive; they represent a major health hazard. Mold adversely affects physical health and behavior in ways that are at times irremediable. Dust carries dust mites that generate large amounts of excrement contributing to sinus problems and infections. Dust mites may contribute to skin problems and other imbalances such as a compromised immune system. Dwellers of a chaotic space are usually semi-unconscious or clueless. They live mostly in quasi-survival mode.

Because dwellers of this type are somehow semi-unconscious or semi-clueless are likely to have a cynical side that brings them a false sense of control over their situation. Such people are also likely to have trouble creating or managing healthy boundaries. These dwellers are also prone to be controlled by the dwellers seen above as types 1 and 2; this happens mostly due to financial issues; chaotic people are not always capable of handling their financial affairs very effectively. With these people, there seems to be a dominant factor that contributes to the main causes of dysfunction in their lives: they abuse drugs or alcohol. Besides their innate addictive nature, such people may also be anally retentive, which causes them to be compulsive hoarders and continuously fill their space up with junk they cannot control. In some cases, the junk takes most of their living space, leaving them feeling stifled, frustrated, cramped, and depressed. Because these people do not feel that they have total control over their lives, they leave the mess unattended and ever expanding. They are busy watching TV, their ultimate distraction.

Very often, mold is such a powerful intoxicant in maladjusted people's lives that they both become unified as they live together day-by-day. Two interesting facts occur with mold issues:

1.	People living in mold-infested dwellings are usually not aware of the mold smell. They are so used to living with mold, their sense of smell has developed some form of resistance to it; such people have an impaired sense of smell that cannot detect the mold scent. When you walk in mold infested homes, you can smell the mildew immediately, but the dwellers cannot; the mold is an intrinsic part of their lives. They walk around with their skin, hair, and clothing smelling musty; these people often complain of frequent respiratory infections but will resist cleaning the mold. They prefer to go into denial when they are told about the mold. Usually, these people's car is also infected with mold; they sit in their car a fair amount of the time and transport it from the dwelling to the car. Cars can also have their own unaddressed mold issues.

2. Mold may be affecting a chaotic dwellers' brain to the extent that their cognitive faculties are impaired. They may often misplace or even lose their telephone and be out of touch with others for extended periods of time. The cognitive impairment may also cause such people to go into denial of their issue. That is one of the reasons why some dwellers living with mold may argue for the harmlessness of the mold; some may deny its existence. Some mold-affected people defend and protect the mold because they have become addicted to it. Some may attack anyone who offers to help get rid of it. Because the chaotic type of person is disoriented, virtually unconscious, or clueless, they are at risk of mental dysfunction. That can cause them to be a danger to themselves and others. Many people of this dysfunctional type are institutionalized.

## 4.	Dweller with a dysfunctional concept of personal space

Personal traits:
This category of people features either counter-cultural types of individuals or some derelicts who appear to have abandoned their body. Their mind also seems to have given up on itself. For these dysfunctional individuals, a brick-and-mortar dwelling is optional; sometimes a vehicle, a spot on the beach or a street corner will serve as dwelling for them. In general, when this situation

persists long-term, it indicates that these people are not functional members of society. They might not quite be able to contribute to the process of evolution. They may have started their life as functional people, and for some traumatic reason, have come to a state of incapacitation or personal invalidation. Even though some of these people may be very intelligent, they are not capable of supporting themselves and more often than not, are a public charge. If these people are industrious, it is usually with activities that are not really productive or life changing. This type of person is very frustrated with the feeling of being stuck and going nowhere in life. Often, they are devoid of the concept of healthy shame, therefore have no healthy boundaries.

This type of person may be plagued by learning disabilities that are sometimes caused by drugs, alcohol, malnutrition, environmental challenges. They may suffer the shock of family violence and abuse, abandonment, childhood trauma and also genetic defects. Sometimes, many of such people seem to have some form of predilection for trash and filth. They are incapable of managing waste properly. Their body care is negligible to non-existent. In many cases, this type of person adopts a pet or several pets that soon end up being neglected or abused, just like their owner. No one can give what they do not have; dysfunctional people cannot provide to other beings the care they do not give to themselves.

Dysfunctional people can be environmentally bio-hazardous. Such individuals often harbor a pronounced mildew smell – and oftentimes a stale cigarettes smell -- that seems to linger wherever they go. Their hair, nails, and skin are usually discolored by filth. Some of these individuals can be very bright and articulate, and may even have come from decent families, however, they are utterly unable to get a handle on their life because of intrinsic psychological damage mostly due to chemical imbalances or mismanaged trauma. These people are often in trouble with the law and there is perpetual drama in their lives. They have been so accustomed to the state of drama that for them, on some level, it is more the norm than the exception. On the hierarchy of human needs, this type of dweller is in a dire survival mode. Their level of awareness indicates that they are virtually unconscious or mostly clueless.

<u>**Challenges:**</u>
This type of person is prone to serious mental illness, infectious diseases along with sinus, lungs and skin problems caused by fungi and parasites. There is a major connection between fungi and cancer. Eventually this type of dweller may develop additional problems in the form of diabetes and other degenerative conditions such as heart disease. In Chinese Medicine, heart health is directly dependent on lung function. This type of person is also prone to confusion, brain fog, and all types of accidents. Mold and mildew account for brain fog in countless people. It is not uncommon to see affected people walking around in tattered clothes, carrying on a heated conversation with themselves. This is a sign of severe malnutrition and deficiencies affecting the brain, particularly if the person is also affected by addictions, besides malnutrition.

The problem with institutionalization

Institutionalization does not necessarily address the root causes of social issues. By focusing on managing the effects of trauma through harsh punishment, fear, coercion, chemical drugs therapy or mechanistic intervention, depending on the institution, the process of institutionalization perpetuates social problems. For instance, serial offenders may be affected by chemical imbalances. Such imbalances may be caused by hard-to-detect microorganisms deteriorating their brain if they have been on a junk food diet and illicit drugs for prolonged amounts of time. This, and countless other factors such as genetic predispositions, sexually transmitted diseases, environmental damage, an untrained character, negative vibrational frequencies, and spiritual bankruptcy can add to existing high levels of toxicity. This combination can yield a defective human that is more malignant than useful to society. The utilization of fear and severe punishment to memorialize the handling of cases that are chosen to serve as a deterrent to other offenders is the norm in the correctional and institutional businesses. In spite of ample correction, crime or dysfunction does not seem to be on a noticeable downward trend. Besides correction, it would benefit institutions to investigate other unexplored underlying causes of dysfunction in humans, namely: environmental, emotional, vibrational, and spiritual.   An effort in the direction of addressing unexplored underlying causes is likely to contribute to rehabilitation instead of the current pattern of stagnation, recidivism, and annihilation.

> *"The fact that the mind rules the body is, in spite of its*
> *neglect by biology and medicine, the most fundamental fact*
> *which we know about the process of life."*

> ~ Franz Alexander

We live our life is a reflection of how we think

Sometimes, it is easy to detect certain traits in individuals. They allow us to know what type of behaviors to expect from them, and knowing their character is always a valuable experience. In most cases, it is the smallest clues that can provide some vital information. In general, how people do anything is how they end up doing everything.

Whether people are operating within the ruling class, the investing class, the working class, or the public charge class, each person seems to carry various positive traits as well as dysfunctional traits. Each trait helps form the character of the different types of persons mentioned above; each type of person has a different concept of personal space which contributes to the complexity of societal structures. What makes some people of types 3 and 4 less subjected to living in adverse condition is their accessibility to personal, family, or public funds. Usually, the assistance of family members that are able to care for them is vital, if they are not institutionalized. The commonality with all types is how they live their life in a certain way relating to their state of mind. The point is that at times, it is very hard to make those people understand the necessity of getting them to run their life in an environmentally sound way by taking responsibility for themselves. The more toxic people are, the more difficult it is for them to take responsibility for their life.

Because our Earth is an incubator for different species placed in it for evolution through adaptation and survival, not one of the types of people mentioned above is to be misconstrued as perfect or ideal. Each type of person, regardless of which class they belong to, comes with a variety of well-intentioned and humanitarian people, but also other categories of people who prove to be assassins, racists, criminals, bigots, political and religious fanatics. All of them are looking to make sense of their own life, in their own ways. Some are well-meaning but misguided which makes them an unfortunate waste of potential. They also all have one thing in common: they are toxic, in various degrees. The more toxic people are, the more problematic their personality and behaviors are. Some people may live an exemplary, well adjusted life, however, they may still exhibit toxic traits: they are not exempt from carrying toxic genetic material passed down to them from several if not all generations. The cornerstone in healing maladjustment is the awareness of complex layers of causality. Once awareness is established, one can work on different energetic levels to bring corrections.

The constant in all types of home dwellers is the same: how one lives is a mirror image of how one's mind works. It is primordial to detoxify one's home, work space, vehicle(s), and person on all levels if one is to reach optimum wellness. Detoxification also extends itself to the level of relationships. It is toxic people who make a relationship toxic because of the toxic attitudes that are involved.

You can tell when someone is not handling stress effectively by the way they systematically trash their living space, office, and car. More often than not, they also trash public places and other people's space, the same way they trash their own space. When the mind is in turmoil, body language screams it. Facts speak louder than words. Many people with PTSD issues end up with not just excessive clutter in their space but also a need to keep things constantly disorganized around them. If they were functioning within a rigidly organized structure at the time of the trauma that caused the PTSD, they will systematically re-arrange their surroundings to be the opposite of the rigid structure that painfully lingers in their memory.

Regardless of how comfortable a maladjusted person may feel in their life, they are not serving the world or themselves properly if they are not capable of addressing the issue of toxicity.

It is not unusual to see people show distress when someone suggests they make lifestyle changes in order to change their health. We are creatures of habit and even in bad habits some people take comfort. Our society is structured in such a way that most average people are:
- Given just enough education to be good employees but not necessary outstanding leaders.
- Paid just enough money to function above revolution level but not in financial freedom.
- Indoctrinated just enough to be obedient to powers that exert control through fear and intimidation but not empowered enough to know that a creative force exists within them.

Because there are no isolated structures, everything we think, feel, say, and do contributes to the current construct of our lives and our patterns; we can also choose to be more mindful of how we move through the evolutionary scale if we are to make our passage on this earth a constructive experience for the environment, humanity, and ourselves.

Maslow's Hierarchy of Needs

Maslow's Hierarchy of Human Needs is a theory presented by Abraham Maslow to categorize human needs and demonstrate that their fulfillment relates to people's developmental stages.

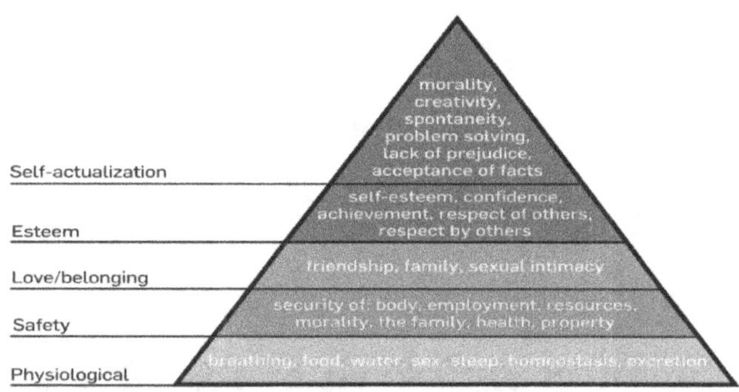

Source: commons.wikimedia.org

This scale addresses humankind's main lifestyle-related matters in a simple but visionary way. It shows where people may be stuck and how their behavior, beliefs, and personal construct contribute to the life they create for themselves.

For example, someone who is stuck at the physiological level may have a preoccupation with the most basic survival needs of humans such as food, shelter, sex, and excretion. A person trapped in this stage is not going to be interested in matters that involve self-achievement, morality, or other paradigms from the self-esteem and self-actualization levels. Also people who attempt to express their creativity – which is in the domain of self-actualization -- but do not have their physiological needs for food and shelter met end up struggling as starving artists. One stage must be properly mastered before one can reach the higher echelons. Other people may be stuck at the level of safety and are too preoccupied with work and productivity to learn how to express love. These people are more capable of functioning at the level of sex, a more primary and basic human need. Love requires a higher level of personal development to function by.

Regarding the hierarchy of needs, the pyramid may also serve to correlate levels of toxicity in proportion to the different stages where individuals fit.

For levity:

Five signs that you're getting old:
1. *You buy a compass to move around in the house.*
2. *You're proud of your lawn mower.*
3. *You would rather work than stay home sick.*
4. *People call you at 9:00 PM and ask: "Did I wake you up?"*
5. *You know what the word 'equity' means.*

Chapter 4

Different Levels of Toxicity

*"For the poison of hatred seated near the heart doubles the burden for the one who suffers the disease;
he is burdened with his own sorrow and groans on seeing another's happiness."*

~ Aeschylus

It is undeniable that we all live in a toxic world where almost everything that is needed for survival is *weaponized*. From the air we breathe, the water we drink, the food we eat, the medicines we take, to the thoughts we process, toxicity is ubiquitous and can be overwhelming.

Human life and animal life were not designed to function through excessive toxicity. Any type of toxicity affects humans and animals individually and collectively. It also affects all other types of organisms that exist. Most humans co-depend on animal flesh for survival. Animals are becoming more and more toxic. More humans and animals on our planet are diseased than at any time in history. The population of overweight and obese people, as seen in the preface, is also rising in spite of massive efforts to get the situation under control. The ordeal that people on Earth are facing nowadays is a monumental issue with toxicity. The three main types of toxicity that affect life on our planet are:

Environmental
Physiological
Psychological

If we look at the reasons why people and animals are getting physically and behaviorally more imbalanced, we can understand that the issue of toxicity is major. Because environmental, physiological, and psychological toxicity all overlap, it is imperative that something be done about the issue of toxicity and it is important that it be done now.

Environmental toxicity issues

If you have never seen a river on fire, you cannot fathom the gravity of environmental pollution. Industrial toxins have polluted our environment and adversely affected our eco-system. An imbalance in the eco-system usually means imbalances in humans and animals, as everything is interconnected. Marine animals are suffocating in the oceans due to extreme chemical toxicity; whales and dolphins are beaching themselves ashore because of severe distress; birds are dropping dead in massive numbers; trees are becoming less resistant and falling to their destruction during even the most minor of storms. As seen earlier, the condition of the collective is a result of each individual action taken day after day, year after year, decade after decade, and century after century. Each mindless action leading to the pollution of the planet contributes to compound the toxicity issue. If each human were to think twice before buying another plastic bottle and remember the detriment it eventually causes to the environment, we would already be close to reaching critical mass regarding our efforts to resolve the pollution mess.

Physiological toxicity issues

The most toxic places in the world are in the areas known as megapolises, where life is mainly industrial and where great emphasis is put on the infrastructure for speedy transportation and massive synthetic food production.

Statistics show that California, New York, New Jersey, Pennsylvania, Mississippi, Alaska, and Oregon have higher cancer rates than other states. Most cancers develop in people living in metropolitan areas with a megapolistic infrastructure. In megapolises, one of the main issues is a lack of quality of life, due to large urban agglomerations that necessitate food, lodging, work, schooling, disease care and entertainment. A large number of middle class dwellers of the megapolises feel unhappy and trapped, plagued with allergies, asthma, bodily pain and degenerative illnesses.

The least adjusted inner city dwellers who may have fallen through the cracks exhibit a perfect example of how bodily toxicity and prolonged malnutrition can exert the most detrimental effects on the functioning of the mind and body. Many survivors of extreme megapolistic toxicity are mentally challenged. They do not, or cannot cook, so they have recourse to either the fast food joints or any low quality foodstuff handed over to them. The least fortunate ones raid garbage disposals for whatever scraps they may find. They are sometimes so depleted physically that they have a tendency to walk in a hunched forward or disorganized manner. A lot of them are limping badly. They look disoriented and some of them are talking to themselves. Part of or all of the above is usually due to substance abuse leading to chemical and mental imbalances. While their manner of dressing does not reflect much dignity, their manner of speaking is as deplorable.

.

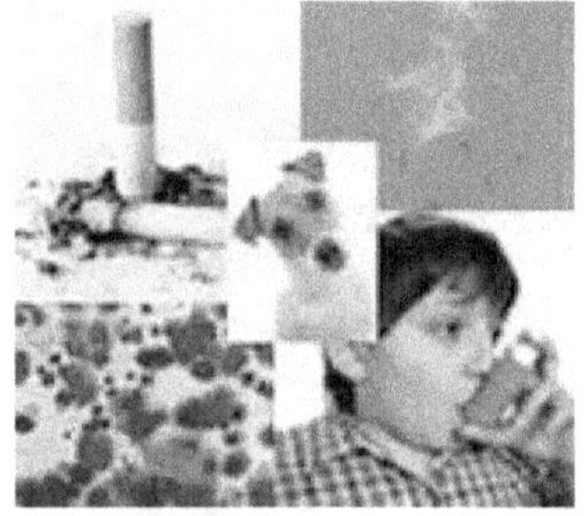

Source: arb.ca.gov

Psychological toxicity issues

When environmental toxicity and physiological toxicity prevail, the psychological body usually gets affected also. There are numerous ways in which psychological toxicity manifests itself. It can take the form of harmful behavior such as aggression, which features a tendency to violate social conventions, leads to truancy, and perpetrates violence. Manifestations of psychological toxicity vary depending on lifestyle, genetics, and levels of toxicity, as well as how long the organism has been exposed to the toxicity and also where one person is positioned on Maslow's Hierarchy of needs. Some of the indicators of psychological toxicity may appear as fear which usually causes: anger, rage, anxiety, depression, guilt, hopelessness, self-destructive tendencies, self-mutilation, self-defacing behavior, attraction to filth and trash, etc. Fear leads to criminality which includes: homicide, domestic violence, terrorism, arson, dilapidation, vandalism, devious entertainment, racial prejudice, pedophilia, addiction to fights and profanity, etc.

"The industrial revolution has tended to produce everywhere great urban masses that seem to be increasingly careless of ethical standards."

~ Irving Babbitt

In many urban areas where the air, food, and water supply contains the frequency of the largest number of pollutants, dwellers also exhibit the highest level of toxic behavior. You may stand in public near someone who comes out of the blue and starts polluting the energy of the air with an excessive use of linguistic improprieties and negativity. There often is overt aggression for no discernible reason. There also is a propensity for extreme cynicism and resistance to behavior modification. It is easy to observe how many maladjusted people are afflicted by a compulsion for profanity, which is also an indication of physiological toxicity combined with psychological toxicity.

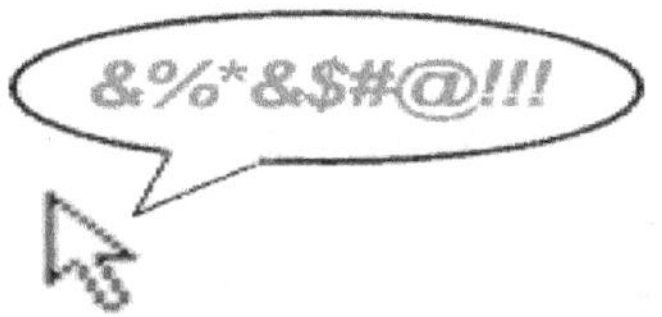

Source: http://kids.niehs.nih.gov/assets/images/p/past5.gif

The pathology of scatology

Our words are a frequency signature of our character and thought processes which relate to the different emotions we process. Far too many people speak in ways that are virtually infectious: every other word is spiked with obscenities. People preoccupied with excretion-related profanity may not even be aware of the behavior. Mark Twain has written: *"Under certain circumstances, profanity provides a relief denied even to prayer."* It is clear that profanity can be used 'under certain circumstances', so, for a sane person, it is not necessarily a habit. In case it is a habit, then the behavior reveals an impulse control disorder. Because of certain individuals' excessive use of obscenity, they leave the impression that they perhaps make a living on a toilet or on their back. Most of the words in their sentences are either scatological or referring to undignified copulation. Compulsive users of scatology-laced language are affected by toxicity. Such people may be stuck at the excretive stage of human growth; people stuck at the excretive stage -- a phase shown in Maslow's Hierarchy of Needs -- are often immature.

Compulsive use of curse words is likely to be a reflection of unaddressed internal toxicity and anally retentive traits. If someone is not moving their bowels regularly, they are likely to have foodstuff rotting in their backed up system. Because the body is a bio-resonant machine, i t releases energetic clues of issues to be addressed internally, particularly when such issues relate to intestinal putrefaction. Because we are what eat, if the food is undigested and rots in our intestines, our mind becomes subconsciously preoccupied with the waste that is overdue for excretion. Additionally, we are our word, so when what is inside of us turns to problematic waste, we verbally express this type of toxicity.

If compulsive potty-mouthed people were put in a position to eat their words, it would be a rather messy proposition! An article on msn.com recently reported by Donna Freedman noted: *"A majority of managers believe that swearing indicates a lack of professionalism, self-control, maturity or intelligence."*

As Dr. Masaru Emoto has demonstrated through his research studies concerning water, words greatly influence matter within our environment. Our words carry wavelengths of frequencies. We create our reality through the frequency of our words. Because everything is related to frequencies, if we dwell more on the low frequency side, our environment can also be contaminated with negative wavelengths. Lower frequencies have longer wavelengths than higher frequencies, and that is probably why it is easier for most humans to resonate with lower frequencies than it is for high frequencies that are in general more beneficial.

Our spoken word is a reflection of our level of consciousness. Humans are an energetic creation of consciousness, and the process of creation involves the spoken word. When we are at integrity with our word and do as we say, we are in alignment with truth. Our word is our seal and our bond. When we fail to be at integrity with our word and use it for improprieties, we end up creating inner guilt, which is a toxic emotion.

The pathology of static behavior

Some people are virtually unable to work with paradigm shifts, regardless of the soundness of the shift. It may have something to do with aging, fear, mainstream indoctrination, or the inability to process new information –   which is also one of the many symptoms of PTSD. The irrationality of static behavior resides in the fact that the affected people know that their behavior is harming them but they continue to behave in ways that perpetuate the harm.

One can be made aware of conditions that require precautions and have the wisdom to adapt. For instance, if you advise your family: "It is snowing now, so wear your snow boots, heavy coat, and hat before going out." In most cases, the forewarned family members will act upon the advisory and the advice may not need to be repeated. So why is it that some people resist or ignore advisory when you repeatedly make them aware of:

- The dangers of eating a late dinner and/or avoiding breakfast.
- The counter-productivity of buying and carrying heavy stacks of bottled water reported by the EPA to be no better than tap. Bottled water may be laced with phthalates, Bisphenol-A, and other contaminants. Some bottled water is acidifying to the body and costs a lot more than a water filter that lasts a lifetime.
- The foolishness of eating or drinking for taste versus health benefits.
- The high toxicity of the top 10 obesity-causing foods.
- The harmful effects of not recycling and reusing.

When people perceive change as a threat, they resist it and remain static. The way they have done things is the way they are likely to keep doing them. Some people change only under a major threat such as death, prison, or going to hell. A person who has neither enough knowledge to lead nor enough sense to follow is a danger to themselves.

For levity:

Q. "Why did New Jersey get all the toxic waste and California all the lawyers?"
A. "Because New Jersey got to pick first."

~ Anon

Part I

ENVIRONMENTAL TOXICITY

Chapter 5

Causes and Effects of Environmental Toxicity

"I thought about the current contamination of beaches, raw sewage spilling into oceans and streams, the hole in the ozone, forests being stripped, the toxic-waste dumps, the merry plunder of mankind added to the drought and the famine that nature dishes up annually as a matter of course. It's hard to know what's actually going to get us first."

~ Sue Grafton

There is compelling evidence indicating that environmental toxicity adversely affects physical and behavioral health. Environmental bio-hazards affecting humans and animals come in the form of stressors that have various sources and reasons for being in the environment.

Criteria of environmental toxicity

It affects the planet and all of its life forms. It is caused mostly by dumping, chemical pollution, improper disposal of industrial waste, radiation by-products, petrochemicals, lead, pesticides, mercury, cadmium, chemtrails, plastics, noise pollution, electromagnetic pollution, etc. There is compelling evidence indicating that environmental pollution contributes to many diseases in humans and animals. Scientists have shown that environmental toxicity is also related to the disappearance of certain a n i m a l species plus the drying up of the earth's bodies of water.

Air pollution

Back in 2001, the EPA released studies showing that 36 people out of one million will get cancer from exposure to the air in America. From nanoparticles of chemical pollutants to chemtrails, mold spores, out-of-control pollen, and countless other organisms, the air we breathe can be very toxic depending on the areas where we live. Some areas are more polluted than others, and understandably, megapolises are the most polluted of all areas. Thanks to the Clean Air Act, some efforts are being made to reduce air pollution. With the propagation of eco-friendly vehicles, there will be more progress.

Water pollution

Most of our waterbeds are contaminated with environmental toxins, plastics, pharmaceutical by-products, and all sorts of contaminants. Bottled water, because it is not subjected to industry regulations is not necessarily a better choice for water consumption than tap water. In 1969, the Cuyahoga River in Cleveland caught on fire due to excessive man-made pollution from hazardous chemicals dumped into it. This caused new regulations to be passed in order to curb excessive water pollution. Nowadays, our waters are polluted in ways that are hazardous to human and animal health. This knowledge has motivated the bottled water industry to offer solutions in the form of packaged water. Now that just about everyone is buying stacks of bottled water, we are facing environmental pollution. People not knowing that plastic bottles litter the environment and take at least one thousand years to bio-degrade. Countless people are also not aware that bottled water has a hazardous side to it since phthalates and Bisphenol-A (BPA), chemicals found in the plastic, leach into the water and cause harmful side effects known as hormonal imbalances and degenerative diseases such as cancer.

Soil pollution

It is related not only to air and water pollution but also to chemical pollution and the dumping of toxic products, pesticides, herbicides, and other toxic products. A lot of the soil pollution comes from plastics of different grades. Plastic dumping is a huge issue. Many people overuse products that are bottled or packaged in plastics but do not properly recycle the waste that ends up littering the environment in very harmful ways.

Electromagnetic pollution

In the environment, electromagnetic pollution may come from high voltage electric fields, power lines, and miscellaneous aerosol pollutants. Electromagnetic pollution is associated with electromagnetic radiation which has been found to be responsible for DNA damage and degenerative illnesses such as cancer, Alzheimer's Disease, etc.

Electromagnetic pollution involves what is known as "dirty electricity" in the form of dangerous electromagnetic fields (EMF) that have been found to cause cancer, leukemia, and other woes. Wherever there are appliances such as television transmitters, radio transmitters, microwave ovens, toaster ovens, refrigerators, hair dryers, electronic devices such as cell phones, computers, and all types of portable electronic devices, there is electromagnetic pollution. One can also receive a significant dose of electromagnetic pollution just by riding in a car or traveling by air, rail, or water. The frequency level of the various electromagnetic fields determines how hazardous the exposure can be.

Here is an excerpt from an article by Walter Last explaining the subject matter:
> *"Strong electromagnetic fields (EMFs) of about 50 to 60 cycles per second (hertz, or Hz) and the related electromagnetic radiation (EMR) are harmful to us. Long-term exposure may aggravate any existing health problems or diseases and may cause or intensify especially lack of energy or fatigue, irritability, aggression, hyperactivity, sleep disorders and emotional instability. Increasing numbers of individuals are becoming hypersensitive to EMR; many can feel the electricity going through the body a chronic exposure to high levels of EMR, especially while asleep, is a constant drain on our vitality. It creates chronic stress, which interferes with the regeneration and healing that normally takes place during a good night's sleep. You may compare it to always swimming against a strong current and this may well make the difference between recovering from a serious disease and succumbing to it."*

For more information on health issues due to electricity and many case reports, see www.emrsafety.8m.net.

Dumping

It happens worldwide and has to do with the exportation of waste – mostly industrial, and sometimes hazardous -- to areas with more lax standards about waste disposal and recycling. It contaminates the waters, the soil, and eventually the air. Dumping occurs:

a. On the land – The toxic waste can contaminate the soil.
b. In the ocean – Contributing to oxygen depletion and the death of marine animals.

Dumping causes wild life to suffer from all sorts of diseases and genetic mutations before dying. It has dire repercussions on the humans who eat animals, drink contaminated water, and eat food from the contaminated soil.

Chemical pollution

It is ubiquitous and the cause of many diseases and deaths in humans, marine life, wild life, and the destruction of bodies of water. It includes:

1. Pesticides

They are designed to kill animal species considered to be in the category of pests. Pesticides, just like herbicides, do what they are designed to do: kill. The word 'cide' is defined in the dictionary as: *"A learned borrowing from Latin meaning 'killer', or act of killing"*. What is also an important point to remember is that pesticides indiscriminately kill animals and humans alike. All that matters is the degree of exposure in terms of dosage, intensity, and duration. There are different grades of pesticides and all of them are harmful. Pesticides get released in the waterbeds and leave residues on the soil and grass. They take a long time to biodegrade, and become neutralized. They start breaking down after application, but their half-life is in average 60 days. The half-life of DDT is 15 years in the soil. Small colorful flags planted in grassy areas usually indicate recent pesticides application and what grade of pesticides has been sprayed over the grass.

2. Herbicides

They are commonly called 'weed killers' and are created to kill plant species that are regarded as 'pesky'. Such weeds can be: dandelion (considered to be a useful blood purifier in herbal medicine), purslane (known to be a very nutritious legume), and a large variety of other plants of the weeds category. For those who doubt the harmful properties of herbicides in humans, it will be an eye opener to check a particular type of herbicide known as Agent Orange. In the following link, one can read an article published on CNN.com revealing how Agent Orange is still causing congenital deformities in babies in Asia, years after their parents were exposed to the substance. http://www.cnn.com/2012/08/10/world/asia/vietnam-us-agent-orange/index.html

3. Embalming ingredients

They are utilized to embalm corpses and eventually end up in the waterbeds and soil. Formaldehyde is one of the products used for that purpose. Quarternium-15 is a quarternary ammonium salt that has been said to have carcinogenic properties. It is found in many personal care products. Quarternium-15 releases the largest amount of free formaldehyde when compared to other FRP (Maier et al 2009). Funeral home operators have reported that there is so much overuse of artificial preservatives in the food supply and personal care products that nowadays, human corpses require 30% less embalming than thirty years ago.

4. Radiation by-products

They are used by the medical profession for the chemical treatment of diseases.

5. Fuel additives

They are in gasoline, and their very volatile nature makes them extremely absorbable by human and animal tissues. Repeated exposure or inhalation of fuel additives has been found to be responsible for health problems.

6. Volatile Organic Compounds (VOCs)

They are known as organic chemicals that are pervasive and have a high vapor pressure at room temperature. They have been found to be hazardous to human life, animal life, and the environment. The following chemicals have been classified within the category of VOCs: chlorofluorocarbons, benzene, methyl chloride, perchloethylene, etc.

7. Carbon Dioxide Emissions

Carbon dioxide (CO_2) is the most major source of heat-trapping gas emitted in the environment through human activities. It is a toxic, poisonous gas. Its excessive emissions have been a reason for concern because it is believed to be responsible for climate change issues, and the greenhouse effect that is associated with global warming. Nowadays, the trees on earth, which normally are designed to filter the air, are demonstrating a lesser ability to reduce CO_2 emissions.

Based on EPA statistics, CO2 emissions are produced mostly by electricity generation (38%), fossil fuel-based transportation (ground, air, and marine) (31%), industrial activity, mainly in the domain of the production of chemicals (14%), residential and commercial activity (10%), and non-fossil fuel combustion (6%).

Synthetic fertilizers a r e u s e d for farming and cattle raising. Cow's flatulence contributes to excess methane gas production because of excessive cow burping. The way cows are raised for meat production is responsible for elevated carbon dioxide emissions. Methane gas is associated with CO_2 production. In today's times, the world's population is eating more meat than perhaps necessary. The higher demand for meat causes a n industry response for larger supply. Even though meat is nourishing, it is also intoxicating for the tissues. It takes a lot of CO_2 producing energy to raise grain-fed cows compared to grass-fed cows. The U.N. Food and Agriculture Organization reported in 2006 that 18% of the world's man-made greenhouse gas production was due to livestock. Elevated amounts of carbon dioxide (CO_2) in the blood are indicative of health issues and an imbalance with oxygen.

8. Chemtrails

They are as their name implies: chemical trails. They involve the spraying of toxic chemicals in our atmosphere. They are different from condensation trails (contrails). They presumably help to control weather patterns and create an atmosphere that will support electromagnetic waves as well as ground-based, electromagnetic field oscillators. Research has shown that the process involves spraying aluminum oxide and barium powder, among many other toxic chemicals. These toxic chemicals are responsible for illnesses, such as Alzheimer's Disease incurred when excess aluminum is stored in the body. There have been reports of new types of respiratory illnesses affecting the population. Incidentally, such reports have been correlating with the advent of chemtrails.

9. Petrochemicals

They are derived from petroleum that is used to manufacture plastics. They are present in almost everything: hair and skin care products, cleaning products, medical care products, and food.

Many people use plastic bottles then throw away the empty containers that some communities do not always properly recycle. Tremendous quantities of plastic bottles and containers end up on the shores, in the ocean, in other bodies of water, and in the soil. Plastic waste causes so much pollution that in the heavily industrialized areas of the planet, it is basically uncontrollable. Plastic is so durable that it takes at least one thousand years to start biodegrading. When plastics and other toxic materials are burned, the fumes contaminate the air and all life forms that breathe the air. Plastic by-products represent a major health hazard in people and animals due to the endocrinological issues they cause. Some of the main known dangerous chemicals found in plastic water bottles are:

    a. Phthalates
    b. Bisphenol-A (BPA)

The following is a section of an abstract on an updated review of the side effects of environmental hazards such as pesticides and industrial chemicals:

For the last 40 y, substantial evidence has surfaced on the hormone-like effects of environmental chemicals such as pesticides and industrial chemicals in wildlife and humans. The endocrine and reproductive effects of these chemicals are believed to be due to their ability to: (1) mimic the effect of endogenous hormones, (2) antagonize the effect of endogenous hormones, (3) disrupt the synthesis and metabolism of endogenous hormones, and (4) disrupt the synthesis and metabolism of hormone receptors. The discovery of hormone-like activity of these chemicals occurred long after they were released into the environment. Aviation crop dusters handling DDT were found to have reduced sperm counts, and workers at a plant producing the insecticide kepone were reported to have lost their libido, became impotent and had low sperm counts. Subsequently, experiments conducted in lab animals demonstrated unambiguously the estrogenic activity of these pesticides. Man-made compounds used in the manufacture of plastics were accidentally found to be estrogenic because they fouled experiments conducted in laboratories studying natural estrogens. For example, polystyrene tubes released nonylphenol, and polycarbonate flasks released bisphenol-A. Alkylphenols are used in the synthesis of detergents (alkylphenol polyethoxylates) and as antioxidants. These detergents are not estrogenic; however, upon degradation during sewage treatment they may release estrogenic alkylphenols. The surfactant nonoxynol is used as intravaginal spermicide and condom lubricant. When administered to lab animals it is metabolized to free nonylphenol. Bisphenol-A was found to contaminate the contents of canned foods; these tin cans are lined with lacquers such as polycarbonate.

Countless research studies have shown that Phthalates and BPA cause DNA damage, and adversely affect bodily organs in humans and animals; moreover, they also represent a hazard for the soil and bodies of water.

Issues with phthalates and bisphenol-A (BPA)

They are chemical compounds added to plastics by manufacturers of plastic products to make plastics more durable and flexible. The are found in just about everything, in plastic water bottles, plastic containers of food, cosmetics, personal care products, children's toys, backpacks, footwear, accessories, and much, much more. Scientific research studies show that phthalates and BPA contribute to:

- cancer and other degenerative diseases in humans.
- endocrine dysfunctions.
- gender-bender issues.
- xenoestrogens production in humans and animals, male and female.

1. In males: phthalates and BPA account for excessive body fat production, prostate problems, breast overgrowth, higher voice pitch, shrinking of the penis, erectile dysfunction, low sperm count, etc. High estrogen levels in men equates low testosterones production.

   Never before in human history have men been so desperate to enlarge their penis. A good look at popular magazines that cater to the male population shows that there is a huge demand for penile enlargement. The demand seems pressing and growing. Most -- and perhaps all -- buyers of penile enlargement products are routinely drinking toxic bottled water. They have not yet become aware that phthalates and Bisphenol-A contribute to the shrinking of male reproductive organs.

2. In females: phthalates and BPA also are responsible for excessive body fat production, breast cancer, uterine cancer, reproductive problems, early puberty in girls, etc. All of such woes are due to the overproduction of xenoestrogens.

3. In babies: intoxication starts at conception. Toxic parents contribute to toxic genetic material forming the baby's body. Phthalates are now being found in babies' umbilical cord blood. Toxic baby food and toxic baby products complete the rest of the toxicity cycle. Most baby items are made of plastics:

   - Baby bottles and bottles nipples
   - Pacifiers
   - Teething rings
   - Baby toys, bath toys
   - Baby feeding spoons, cups, and dishes
   - Baby bath, lotion, and powder bottles

4. In animals: the feminization of male fish, a phenomenon that inhibits reproduction therefore decreases the food supply.

10. Inorganic chemicals

They are of different types and uses, for example:

a. Phosphates

Most laundry detergents and household cleaning products have been found to contain phosphates. Other items that harbor phosphates are: paint, personal care products, and even processed packaged food. Phosphates are inorganic chemical compounds containing phosphorus. Many rivers and streams have been drying up due to excessive amounts of phosphates in the water supply.

b. Chlorine

Even though chlorine is a necessity that municipalities routinely use for water disinfection, it also has side effects. In institutions, commercial venues and households, chlorine is used for cleaning, disinfection, and bleaching. Even in extremely diluted amounts, prolonged and frequent use for water disinfection, showering and swimming poses risks of cancer and health issues such as thyroid dysfunction leading to excess weight gain.

c. Nitrogen

It is often used in crop fertilization and for other industrial purposes. Sulfites and sulfates that derive from nitrogen are heavily used in the personal care industry for the manufacture of hair care and skin care products. Sodium lauryl sulfate and sodium laurel sulfate (SLS) have been found to be carcinogenic.

d. Mercury

A chemical element used in dentistry and other industries. Its vapors can cause very serious health problems. It used to be an essential part of thermometers but has been banned for a few years now. Mercury also enters in the manufacture of some compact fluorescent light bulbs.

e. Cadmium

A chemical element found in batteries. When improperly disposed of, cadmium makes its way into the waterbed and soil, adversely affecting our food production.

f. Lithium

When lithium batteries are improperly disposed of, the soil and water do become contaminated by this heavy metal. Even though in micro doses, bioavailable types of lithium are useful as medicine, excessive exposure to lithium leaking from batteries in the environment can cause toxic overload and eventually overtax the body.

g. Lead

It is a highly toxic metal found on the earth's crust and also in man-made items. The main problem with man-made items is their improper disposal or recycling. Exposure to lead has caused numerous types of illnesses, both physical and behavioral. It has been responsible for genetic damage and birth defects. Lead is included in paint, cellular phones batteries, certain types of glass, some cosmetics (particularly lipsticks, foundation, and eye shadow). Lead is also present in some electrical cords and wiring materials. Batteries represent 80 percent of the lead supply worldwide; lead emissions are 20 times higher in Mexico than in the US.

In the 1980s, New York City was one of the most polluted places in the United States. There was an extremely high rate of littering, lowering IQs, and imprisonment due to increasing criminality, violence, and rebellious behavior. There was an overwhelming amount of graffiti in the infrastructure, particularly the subways, bridges, overpasses, and walls. Then, in the mid-to-late 1980s after clinical studies revealed the connection between lead paint in homes and the prevalence of vandalism due to mental dysfunction, the officials of the city initiated lead-based paint control. Some time after the use of lead became regulated, the rate of vandalism, mental illness, criminality and imprisonment significantly decreased.

Some studies have shown that Houston, Texas has high levels of environmental pollutants and also registers a prevalence of illiteracy, learning disabilities, and a high rate of imprisonment of young men due to criminality. New York's Mayor, Michael Bloomberg, has at some point pioneered the banning of the overuse of soft drinks. The bitter news is: soft drinks have played a major role in the epidemic of overweight, obese, and diabetic people.

Noise pollution

It is a major problem in mega cities, especially in the inner cities. There are different types of noise that range from industrial to harmful sonic frequencies, some of which are not always detectable. Noise pollution is everywhere, however it is much more prevalent in high density areas such as the cities that never sleep. Noise affects our sense of hearing and also our sanity.

Most of the detectable noise usually comes from: engines, heavy machinery, all types of vehicles, landing and ascending aircraft, trains, police vehicles, fire trucks, and ambulance sirens, loud sounds from broken car and motorcycle mufflers, loud radio playing, people, barking dogs, etc. It is always an unpleasant experience to be awakened in the middle of the night by loud, alarming noises. In the inner cities in particular, where loud gun shots are commonplace, there is additional stress that assaults the mind and adversely affects hearing and peace of mind. Individuals who live near an airport, a highway, or railroad tracks can be subjected to severe noise pollution. In general, people living in areas of high population density are more likely to be the recipients of abuse from noise pollution than those living in rural areas.

Frequent and prolonged exposure to sounds higher than 85 decibels has contributed to hearing loss. Noise pollution leads to psychological disturbances, sleep disorders that eventually contribute to metabolic issues, premature aging, hearing loss, degenerative diseases and death.

People living in toxic metropolitan areas are often particularly affected not only by the areas' intrinsic pollution, but also by the prevailing energetic disconnection between humans and the Earth. Even though the number of harmful elements in the environment is virtually limitless, the following list categorizes some of the most major hazards.

ENVIRONMENTAL STRESSORS

Stressors types	Causes of Toxicity	Effects of Toxicity
Toxic air	Industrial pollution, discharge from petroleum refineries, toxic fumes from incineration of municipal trash, chemtrails, ozone, aerosols, chlorofluorocarbons (CFCs), asbestos, radon, carbon monoxide, carbon dioxide (CO2), aluminum oxide, radionuclides, out of control pollen, toxic furniture material, etc	Increased risk of cancer, lungs diseases, allergies, skin problems, liver, kidney, problems, eye, noise, throat discomfort, brain fog, oxygen depletion in the blood, premature aging, etc.
Toxic water	Microorganisms (cryptosporidium, Giardia lamblia, legionella, coliform => including fecal coliform and E. Coli bacteria), turbidity, viruses, disinfectants, disinfection by-products, inorganic chemicals, organic volatile compounds (VOCs), trihalomethanes, chlorine, arsenic, asbestos, barium, cadmium, cyanide, mercury, nitrates, nitrites, benzene, dioxin, heptachlor epoxide, polychlorinated biphenyls (BCBs), styrene, fluoride, aluminum, lead, tetrachloroethylene, toluene, toxaphene, trichlorobenzene, vinyl chloride, xylenes, radium, uranium, organic chemicals, radionuclides, radioactive material, beta particles, photon emitters, etc.	Increased risk of cancer, lungs diseases, liver, kidney, or central nervous system damage, anemia, increase in blood cholesterol, intestinal polyps, increase in blood pressure, intestinal lesions, delays in physical or mental development; ADD/ADHD, learning disabilities, shortness of breath, endocrinological disorders, blue-baby syndrome, numbness, circulatory problems, premature aging, bowel issues, hormonal imbalances, low testosterones production, etc.
Toxic soil	Chemical and industrial dumping, un-recycled plastics, oil spills, overuse of pesticides, herbicides, pharmaceutical by-products, leaching of all kinds of pollutants, etc.	Toxic food supply.
Toxic food	Pesticides, radiation, preservatives, food additives, nano-technology particles, irradiation, free radicals, heavy metals, trans fats, etc.	Illness
Toxic buildings	Asbestos, volatile toxic gases, EMF, etc.	Allergies, cancer, etc.
Noise	Traffic, aircraft, trains, damaged mufflers of cars and motorcycles, alarms, heavy machinery, etc.	Hearing impairments, cognitive issues, neurological disturbances, sleep disorders.
Electromagnetic radiation	Use of cell phones, computers, other electronic devices, TV, microwave ovens, toaster ovens, hair dryers, air travel, train travel, car travel, etc.	Increased risk of cancer, cognitive and behavioral issues, skin diseases, hair loss, genetic mutations, etc.

<u>**Useful resources:**</u>

1. Dr. Mercola :: Electromagnetic pollution report:
   http://articles.mercola.com/sites/articles/archive/2011/02/16/raising-awareness-about-electromagnetic-pollution.aspx
2. Environmental Protection Agency :: Drinking Water Contaminants Report:
   http://water.epa.gov/drink/contaminants/index.cfm
3. Environmental Protection Agency :: Air Pollutants Report: http://www.epa.gov/oar/airpollutants.html
4. LA Times :: Article on carbon dioxide: http://articles.latimes.com/2007/oct/15/opinion/ed-methane15
5. CBS News report :: Phthalates-containing children's items   http://www.cbsnews.com/2300-204_162-10014609-12.html

Issues with environmental littering and garbage overload

The average American produces approximately four pounds of garbage every day and municipalities are having trouble finding out where to put it. There have been attempts to burn garbage and dump it into the ocean, launch it into space, bury it in the soil, insert it in the food supply, footwear, clothing, accessories, etc. A sound and perfected solution has not yet been found. Garbage overload comes with wastefulness that is due to excessive consumerism.

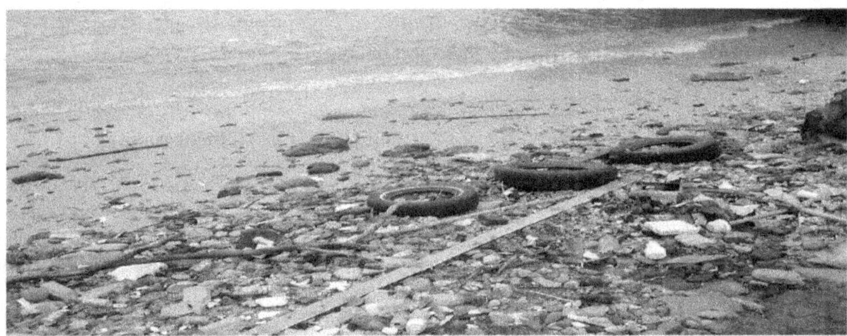

Source: commons.wikimedia.org

People who are not aware of the connection between environmental toxicity and their own state of dis-ease often engage in littering that is a lack of cooperation toward environmental protection. It is akin to vandalism. The general overtone in toxic people's behavior seems to be a focus on neglect and dissonance. A long-term observation of this type of behavior can sensibly lead to the conclusion that most of the behavior is virtually unconscious. A lack of resonance with living in harmony with nature engenders chaos. When people are disconnected from source energy, they are consequently disconnected from each other. Many humans subscribe to the belief that they do not see the need to have any regard for other people's rights and sensibilities. That is one of the reasons why way too many people do not care and litter their own city, home, and vehicles.

Some people have argued that everything that exists on the planet is natural because it originates from nature. Not everything considered natural is healthy however. Plastics originate from the petroleum that is extracted from the earth. Most of them unfortunately also come with irreversible side effects on human and animal health, no matter how natural they are considered to be. Some synthetic foods, such as processed cheese, are often one molecule away from plastic. Since we are what we breathe, eat, drink, feel, hear, see, touch, and think, it is our prerogative to educate ourselves on what comes in contact with our body. The reason for doing that is because toxic pollutants usually have detrimental implications on our health and behaviors.

For levity:

"It's a bad day when the morning news reveals that your home wasn't built on a toxic waste site because... they can't store toxic waste on a native burial ground."

~ Anon

Chapter 6

Solutions to Environmental Toxicity

*"The best way to detoxify is to stop putting toxic things into the body
and depend on its own mechanism."*

~ Dr. Andrew Weil

I. Detoxify

Air

A. To properly filter the pollution out of the air, it is important to secure a quality air filter, especially if one lives in a dense population or wherever air quality is bad. People with allergies, immune depletion, sensitivities, or passive smoking issues can greatly benefit from an air filter.

B. In addition to an air filter, it is recommended to keep in one's space different kinds of plants that are known to filter the air naturally. A NASA Clean Air Study conducted in the 1980s revealed that several plants have air purifying properties. Of course, the plants do take longer than a mechanical air filter to perform, however, they are quite useful while one is waiting for a new filter to be shipped. Plants, in addition to an air filter, work synergistically for maximum benefit. Plants used for indoor air purification are:

1. Bamboo
2. Boston Fern
3. Chinese Evergreen
4. Chrysanthemum
5. Dumb Cane
6. Dwarf Palm
7. Orchid
8. Peace Lily
9. Photos
10. Snake Plant
11. Philodendron
12. Spider Plant

Air filtering plants do have a tendency to collect more dust than others, therefore it is necessary to clean the leaves on a regular basis for the filtration process to be effective.

<u>**Useful resource**</u>:
Wikipedia :: Complete list of air filtering plants: http://en.wikipedia.org/wiki/List_of_air-filtering_plants

Water

A high quality water filter can serve to detoxify the tap and remove contaminants as well as turbidity. Filtering tap water with a good filter before drinking it prevents the accumulation of phthalates and Bisphenol-A in the body. A filter can also put an end to the slavery of buying and carrying stacks of water bottles, an especially hard task if one has back pain. It also prevents environmental littering. Tests have shown that regardless of the brand, most bottled water is no better than tap. Bottled water acidifies the blood, whereas filtered water is more likely to promote a neutral to slightly alkaline pH that is essential to health. An acidic body leads to disease and death. Water accounts for an average of 60% of the body's weight. Since we are what we drink, it is of utmost importance to introduce only the highest quality of water into our system. That is especially valid if we want to have quality health. The US Geological Survey's Water Science School has posted the following data on its website:

> Water is of major importance to all living things; in some organisms, up to 90% of their body weight comes from water. Up to 60% of the human body is water, the brain is composed of 70% water, and the lungs are nearly 90% water. Lean muscle tissue contains about 75% water by weight, as is the brain; body fat contains 10% water and bone has 22% water. About 83% of our blood is water, which helps digest our food, transport waste, and control body temperature. Each day humans must replace 2.4 liters of water, some through drinking and the rest taken by the body from the foods eaten.
>
> According to Dr. Jeffrey Utz, Neuroscience pediatrics, Allegheny University, different people have different percentages of their bodies made up of water. Babies have the most, being born at about 78%. By one year of age, that amount drops to about 65%. In adult men, about 60% of their bodies are water.
> Source: http://ga.water.usgs.gov/edu/propertyyou.html

<u>**Useful resources**</u>:
Sources of quality water purification systems:
1. http://www.multipure.com 1-800-629-9206 – Distributorship #426453
2. http://abetterworld.tv/water-filtration/

Soil

In order to accommodate the need to feed the world's growing population, the agricultural industry has had recourse to industrial methods of growing. Such methods have proven to have a downside that translates into soil depletion that has led to soil erosion and a lessening of the quality of nutrients in the crops. It is possible to grow food in eco-friendly ways that can yield abundant and non-toxic produce. Besides conventional agriculture and organic growing, there are different ways of growing food. Some of them work without chemical fertilizers and without requiring the skills and experience of a professional farmer. They include:

1.   Hydroponic/Aquaponic growing (of plants and fish)
2.   Permaculture
3.   Bio-dynamic growing
4.   Vertical growing

Useful resources:
Sources of bio-dynamic growing systems:
1. Aquaponics: http://www.aquaponicssecrets.org/?hop=pcg111
2. Successful organic gardening: http://www.food4wealth.com/?hop=pcg111
3. DIY Womery: http://0066cbl44wgq2wcj2iv3zcniiy.hop.clickbank.net/

Food

1. Eat organic or pesticides-free, and free-range as much as convenient.
2. Buy your food supply from an organic food cooperative or farmers' market.
3. Grow your own food if possible.
4. Wash all fruits and vegetables thoroughly to remove residues of pesticides, fungicides, chemical or organic fertilizers, and any kind of toxins brought on by insects and parasites.
5. Prepare your own food as much as possible. You have no control over how commercial food is prepared.

How to wash produce

a)   Always wash the produce thoroughly.
b)   Scrub meticulously with baking soda and or diluted peroxide, or mild vegetable soap such as Castile soap. Use a loofah sponge or a brush made of natural fibers.
c)   For green leaf produce, run your fingers all over it, under a steady stream of running water, to remove an slimy film from bacteria and impurities.
d)   Rinse the produce with purified water before consumption.

Why wash produce?

Because produce is in intimate contact with pesticides, fungicides, and herbicides, it is primordial to sanitize it. Produce is also in contact with crawling insects, and predatory animals that usually carry germs, viruses, or venom. During the picking and handling of produce, the laborers who process the produce are an additional source of toxic pollutants. Produce of any type must be thoroughly washed and rinsed before consumption. The reason why it is so very important to rinse the produce with purified water is because using contaminated water is hazardous. When the rinse water has more pollutants than there are on the produce, the action of cleaning the produce is then counterproductive.

Some people think that because their produce is organic, then they do not have to clean it. This belief is faulty for the following reasons:

1)   Even so-called organic produce may harbor some pesticides, herbicides, countless parasites, harmful microorganisms, and other contaminants. Consequently, it is important to be aware that:

> a. It is the percentage of pesticides in the produce that determines the criteria for labeling it as organic. Usually, with 3% pesticides or less, the produce can legally be labeled as organic.

> b. In the fields where some produce is grown, there are no restrooms and sinks. Produce pickers and handlers may not have the opportunity to clean their hands when handling produce.

2)   Proper sanitation always minimizes the risk of diseases from germs.

The following items are non-toxic and can be used safely and beneficially to remove toxic residues on produce:

1. Diluted pure liquid Castile soap – rinse well with purified water after use.

2. Diluted peroxide for 2 to 5 minute soaking – 1 tbsp per quart of pure water then rinse the produce with pure water.

3. Baking soda -- use for scrubbing then rinse with pure water.

4. Fine sea salt -- use as a non-toxic scrubbing agent for produce.

5. Bentonite clay and Diatomaceous Earth -- when properly purified, both can serve as natural cleansing agents for produce with firm surface like carrots, eggplant, etc.

Useful resources:
Bentonite clay :: Contact: wholeness.mission@gmail.com or call (201) 676-0706.
Dr. Carolyn Dean's wellness program :: http://8b60eer57wcq8lc2l50j-june0.hop.clickbank.net/?tid=J9578G87

Plastic products

Plastics offer a huge number of benefits, from waterproofing to the convenience of quick, easy handling, shatter-proof qualities, in addition to effective spill reduction. Plastics are unsurpassed when it comes to the utility of such items as flip caps, squeeze bottles, rain boots, computers, cellular phones, fax machines, medical devices such as catheters, for instance. Regardless of the enormous conveniences of plastics, unfortunately, there is a dangerous side to them. With the exception of food-grade plastic, plastic by-products such as phthalates and Bisphenol-A have been found to have serious side effects on humans and animals alike. To reduce the effects of phthalates, Bisphenol-A, and other plastic-related harmful by-products, replace mainstream plastic products with: glass, stainless steel, ceramic, wood, or other non-toxic, durable material as much as possible.

Teflon

Teflon cooking utensils contain a grade of plastic with particles that can leach into food and contribute to serious health problems. Consider replacing teflon utensils with either:
1. Stainless steel.
2. Cast iron.
3. Ceramic.
4. Glass.
5. 'Green' (eco-friendly), non-stick, cooking utensils.

Plastic cooking items

They are known to be toxic:
1. Plastic ladles, serving spoons, spatulas, and related items.
2. Plastic cutting boards, etc.

One is better off replacing them with items made of stainless steel or ceramic.

Cleaning products

From dishwashing liquids to bathtub cleansing foams, cleaning products can contain harmful petrochemicals that may cause long-term health issues. Replace toxic cleaning products with environmentally-friendly, 'green' products.

"I don't think whole populations are villainous, but Americans are just extraordinarily unaware of all kinds of things. If you live in the middle of that vast continent, with apparently everything your heart could wish for just because you were born there, then why worry? [...] If people lose knowledge, sympathy and understanding of the natural world, they're going to mistreat it and will not ask their politicians to care for it."

~ David Attenborough

Noise

To help control the situation:
1. Wear ear plugs.
2. Wrap a scarf around the ears at bedtime to muffle any type of noise.
3. Wear headphones to play sounds containing embedded therapeutic frequencies.
4. Play soothing background sounds or sound frequencies to counteract the noise.
5. Soundproof the room(s).

II. Practice conscientious hygiene

When it comes to preferences in sanitation, they tell us who is more likely to be a vector and transmitter of toxins, therefore diseases. One of the simplest, yet most self-protective actions is the habit of washing one's hands. Yet, many individuals resist washing their hands before important activities such as eating or providing care to someone else. Hands are carriers of toxins and germs. People contaminate each other by transmitting viruses, harmful bacteria, and parasites to each other, by shaking hands and touching all types of contaminants. Observe people using public restrooms and witness that in average, 70% of men leave without ever washing their hands, compared to 30% of women. It is a nauseating fact, particularly when parents accompanying children are clueless to the point of not knowing anything about sanitation. Some parents do not teach their children that in order to prevent the spread of diseases, they must wash their hands after using a toilet. Since people cannot give what they do not have, a parent who was not taught hygiene cannot pass the useful knowledge to their offspring.

At home:

1. Wash your hands often, especially before preparing and consuming food. Hands are always in contact with something in the awake state. Before and after urinating or defecating, wash your hands with Castile soap. Since you're going to touch toilet paper to wipe yourself, you can decrease the contamination of the paper by washing the hands well. Proper hands sanitation is a multi-step method and here are the specific steps:
   1. Turn the faucet on and wet the hands.
   2. Apply liquid soap on the hands and rub the hands with soap lather for at least 5 seconds. At times, a brush is useful for scrubbing the hands and the areas under the nails.
   3. Rinse the hands under running water until the soap is cleared out.
   4. Take a clean piece of paper towel and turn the faucet off. Your bare hands should not touch the faucet's knob if there are other people using the restroom. Because the un-sanitized hands from other people in the household may touch the faucet, there is a high risk of contamination.
   5. Dry your hands with a clean, dry sheet of paper towel.
   6. Open the restroom door with paper towel. Restroom doors and door knobs are usually contaminated. Paper towels shield the hands from contaminants. To keep the hands clean, shield them from all other door knobs afterwards.

It is basic, but extremely important, to properly sanitize one's hands before preparing and handling food, caring for babies, the elderly, and after handling pets.

2. Close the toilet lid before flushing to prevent toilet water droplets from projecting.

3. Keep toothbrushes inside a closed medicine cabinet or in a sheath to avoid contaminants.

4. Take your shoes off when entering your living quarters. By doing so, you minimize the spread of environmental toxins inside your dwelling. Some of the toxins include:

> a. Pesticides – As seen in the previous chapter , pesticides be can harmful, particularly when overused.

> b. Phthalates –   Such by-products of plastics can be a source of contamination for your hands when handling certain items and even non-plastic ones such as cash register receipts.

> c. Microorganisms, parasites, viruses, harmful bacteria, etc. For example, pigeon droppings are known to carry infectious contaminants.

>> The New York Department of Health and Mental Hygiene's website reports useful information on pigeons as follows:
>>
>> Contact with pigeon droppings may pose a small health risk. Three human diseases are known to be associated with pigeon droppings: histoplasmosis, cryptococcosis, and psittacosis.
>> Source: http://www.nyc.gov/html/doh/html/epi/epi-pigeon.shtml

5. Avoid putting the feet on beds, coffee tables, and desks while shoes or slippers are on. Avoid walking barefoot on carpeting: you risk sharing microorganisms by doing so. Fungus may stay on the carpeting and contaminate people walking on it; other micro-organisms and pollutants from the carpeting may come from pets and pollens.

In public:

1.   In public restrooms:

> 1. Wipe, then cover the toilet seat with clean tissue before sitting.
>
> 2. After using the toilet, thoroughly wash hands and dry them with paper. Hand dryers do not protect one's hands from harmful organisms and may even help spread germs. It is necessary to use clean paper towels to turn public restrooms' faucets on and off, and also open doors. Restrooms that offer a hand-drying machine -- but no paper towels -- are not fully sanitary. Once the hands are dried and then touch the door, the hands may be re-contaminated. The paper towel used to shield the hands is more sanitary than the dryer in public restrooms.
>
> 3. Avoid putting one's purse or other belongings on the floor. Even seemingly clean public restrooms may have particles of fecal matter that can end up on the bottom of purses and bags.

Additional solutions for toxicity prevention and damage control

Ventilate

In some homes, at times indoor air can be a lot more polluted than outdoor air. In this case – and even if in doubt about the air quality - ventilate the place regularly and thoroughly to force pollutants out and renew the oxygen levels.

Plant trees

Green your home, your surroundings and beyond by growing different kinds of plants. Plant as many trees as possible. Greening helps the renewal of oxygen. Use mainly plants that clean and filter the air.

Support environmentally-conscious organizations and causes

Whether they are green landscaping companies, organic food co-ops, green stock brokerage firms, green printing companies, green web hosting companies, make an encouraging statement with your patronage.

Recycle

Even though municipalities have been making an effort to encourage recycling, most people are not up to speed with recycling yet. More of an educational process is required before the masses are able to subconsciously know where and how to dispose of their plastics, what types of plastics to recycle (there are seven of them), how to recycle glass, paper, cardboard, etc., rather than dumping this type of waste material in the garbage can.

Re-use glass, stainless steel and other non-toxic materials

Some food cooperatives are encouraging their patrons to bring their own non-plastic containers to purchase food. There is a lot of merit to this initiative and if more people were to do the same, the population would be well on its way to bringing at least one solution to numerous environmental issues. It makes environmental sense to take the stainless steel canteen to the Chinese food take-out and all other take-out restaurants.

Use eco-friendly laundry products and dishwashing detergents

They are less likely to have the high level of phosphates that have been hazardous to the eco-system.

Buy food and other household necessities in bulk

This solution saves time and effort shopping while it is more economical. It also helps one become conditioned to reuse items that already are in the household, therefore preventing additional purchase of plastic, cardboard and all other types of packaging.

Purchase eco-friendly vehicles

There are different types of eco-friendly vehicles from hybrid cars (that run on battery and fuel) to ones that run on alternative fuel. They are worth acquiring.

Carpool

In different parts of the world, some aware members of ecologically-conscious communities are engaging in carpooling for environmental and economical purposes. Carpooling also fosters a sense of community involvement.

Use eco-friendly buses

More municipalities are using them as of now. They generate fewer emissions.

Buy and use recycled paper goods

There are available in many stores worldwide.

Help curb garbage overload

Food packaging, cloth diapers, unrecyclable items like grease-filled cardboard, all need to have their consumption curbed if municipalities are to get the garbage problem under control and protect the environment.

Practice mindfulness and benevolence

Be aware that your thoughts and emotions affect the environment. Planet Earth is a living organism and on an energetic level, everything we do – including the thoughts and emotions we emit – do affect it. The love and care you put out helps raise planetary frequency at a vibrational level.

Take action toward helping environmental causes

Numerous causes are raising awareness on ecological issues. Get involved.

Use ecofriendly pesticides

Diatomaceous Earth is a clay-like powder that works well to exterminate pesky insects such as roaches, bed bugs, ants, and more.

For levity:

"When I was a boy, the Dead Sea was only sick."

~ Anon

Chapter 7

Detoxification of the Home

"The strength of a nation derives from the integrity of the home."

~ Confucius

If you have ever entered a house to find yourself under the effect of fatigue, irritability, or other discomfort, you might have visited a toxic home... Usually, toxic homes are inhabited by toxic people. Chances are that when you entered that toxic home, there was an excess of: dust, clutter, electromagnetic radiation, emissions from toxic chemicals, radon gas; maybe there were radiator or boiler room issues, sound frequencies radiating from water pipes, steam, or gas pipes, constant loud noises, and anything else that usually affects the human energy field. Moreover, there may have been chaotic furniture arrangement, discordant mismatched colors and patterns, and perhaps illness or disagreement on the premises. Usually a toxic home has the TV on all the time.

You cannot effectively detoxify your physical body or your energetic self, unless your home is cleared from the energetic debris affecting your state of mind and your physical health. A disorganized and untidy home is grounds for depression, high blood pressure, and other issues. No amount of treatment can fully remedy the problem unless you start solving it from the root cause, within your immediate environment. When you clear the home, introduce healing elements to it, e.g. live plants and flowers, and then start taking appropriate measures to detoxify and heal yourself. It will be energy well spent.

The front and / or back entrance, porch, and yard

Possible causes of toxicity:

A toxic home's entrance may exhibit:

1. Toxic plants such as poison ivy that may be growing out of control.

2. Excess pollen shedding from various plants.

3. Old rain water in contact with decaying organic material such as old leaves, planters, and rotting items that may have been affected by different types of mold.

4. Pet dander and pet waste.

Remedies:

1. Remove all old items that are suspected of harboring mold caused by rain, humidity, and moisture.

2. Do a clean sweep.

3. For dusty surface, it is ok to use a regular cloth moistened with a diluted solution of purified water and a few drops of essential oil.

4. For moldy/mildewy surface, spray the whole surface with water containing baking soda. The dilution can be as follows: one quart of water for 1 tablespoon of baking soda. Let the baking soda get completely diluted before pumping to avoid clogging the pump. Baking soda has no known level of toxicity for this cleaning task and can help control mold and fungi. For severe mold infestation, ozonation is a must.

5. As an all-purpose cleaner, dilute six drops of Tea Tree oil in one quart of water and spray the surface to be cleansed or disinfected. Tea Tree oil is antiseptic, antibacterial, and antifungal. It controls mold, fungi, and h a r m f u l micro-organisms. It is pleasantly scented and long lasting. Cedar oil has very similar properties and is likely to be a lot more powerful and pricier. It can also be used as a substitute for Tea Tree oil.

The living room, bedroom, study, and leisure room

Possible causes of toxicity:

1. Dust and contaminants

    Household dust is made of many different types of components: dead skin cells, micro particles of deteriorating vehicles tires, soil particles, dirt, decomposing dead insects carcasses, lint from clothing, bedding, towels, drapes, and carpeting, natural biodegradation of paper, books, leather, etc. Dust carries dust mites because the mites feed off the dust and leave their waste in it.

    Dust mites are potent biological allergens. The main problem with mites is that they generate large amounts of excrement that are a major factor contributing to allergies, respiratory infections, and issues with a compromised immune system, to say the least.

An old couch that is never vacuumed or cleaned may be filled with dust mites, parasites, and microorganisms, especially if there is a couch potato that lies on it often.

2. Pet dander

It can be ubiquitous when pets are present but must be kept under control to prevent or curb symptoms of allergies.

3. Electromagnetic pollution

The living room is an area that is likely to register a lot of electromagnetic radiation, since that is usually where there is a television set. The longer the TV runs, the higher the level of electromagnetic pollution. This can be verified by the larger amount of dust that gathers on the TV set compared to furniture or other surfaces.

To determine the level of radiation, use a Gauss meter that can be purchased at a local hardware store. There are side effects from frequent exposure to any type of radiation. It is a known cause for cancer and leukemia.

4. Decorative items and lifestyle products

Some types of scented candles have been found to contaminate the air and cause respiratory issues due to the phthalates and other synthetic chemicals they contain.

Remedies:

1. Control dust, germs, and contaminants .

    a. First, meticulously remove all dust.

        1. Pay attention to the ventilation ducts that can gather a lot of dust and therefore contaminants.

        2. Do not just brush the dust away with feather dusters: this action only displaces the dust, moving it around from one area to another, and allowing it to access your nostrils and lungs too in the process.

        3. Spray a clean cloth or large piece of paper towel with a solution of: an extremely diluted (one to three drops) tea tree oil, essential oil of lemon, cedar, or eucalyptus in one quart of purified water. Thorough clean all surface with the solution.

4. Wipe surfaces clean and keep wiping until there is no trace of dust.

5. After wiping surfaces, use a more concentrated solution (you can double the amount of essential oils) to disinfect doors, door knobs and other surface.

6. Depending on personal preferences, one can also use eco-friendly commercial disinfectants for surfaces that require disinfection.

Main items to clean:
. Remote control devices (they can be very germy)
. Couches
. Rugs
. Drapes
. Window shades
. All furniture (tall pieces of furniture can hide massive amounts of dust on the top surface)
. Walls
. Ceiling fans
. Lamp shades
. Silk plants
. Live plants (they can collect a lot of dust)
. Decoration
. Old books
. Old shoes
. Appliances (esp. the TV set can attract a lot more dust due to static)
. Door and window frames (particularly the top part where a lot of dust can hide)

b. Vacuum clean thoroughly, especially under the couch(es) and also vacuum the couch(es) all over. Pay special attention to the space along the walls, using the vacuum cleaner hose and suction hard-to-reach areas where dust usually accumulates. The order of the vacuum cleaning process can go as follows:

. Couches
. Carpets
. Rugs
. Ventilation ducts
. Floors
. Lamp shades`
. etc.

c. Disinfect the floor, surfaces, and all door knobs.

d. Radiation control

1. Minimize usage of the TV.

2. Measure the radiation levels with a Gauss meter.

3. Use an anti-radiation device.

4. Explore and play soothing, healing sound frequencies.

5. Place bamboo and other air filtering plants in strategic corners of the room.

6. Position a salt lamp near the bed, dresser, desk, and couch.

Usually, wherever there is a high level of radiation, there is also a lot more dust. Anyone can verify this by observing how much dust appliances such as television sets, fax machines, computers, usually attract.

Salt lamps are made of Himalayan salt crystals that increase the level of negative ions in the indoor air. Negative ions ionize the air to the extent of producing a beneficial effect on health. Inversely, positive ions from appliances cause physical and emotional stress.

The kitchen

Possible causes of toxicity:

They are numerous and some of them are:

1. Toxic air

2. Toxic water

3. Contaminants: dust, mold, mildew, etc.

4. Toxic cleaning products

5. Toxic cookware

6. Toxic housewares

7. Noxious gases

8. Electromagnetic pollution

Toxic homes usually contain cleaning products that are most hazardous to health. It is essential to detoxify. The first step is to identify the hazards. The second step is to take action toward eliminating the hazards. The third step is to replace all hazardous items and systems with health-conscious ones.

a. Toxic air detoxification

The quality of our indoor air depends on the quality of the products we clean surfaces with (for counter tops, appliances, floors, etc.) It is important to detoxify the air by installing an air filter in the room where household members spend the most time.

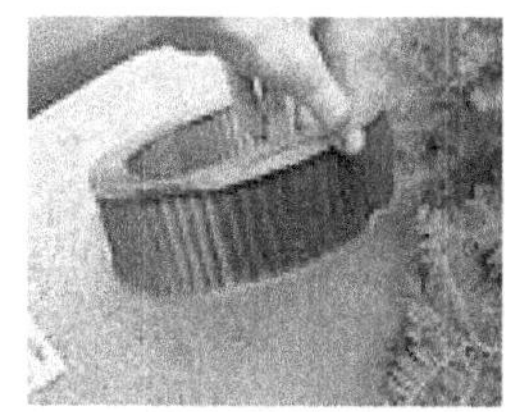

This filter equals $\longrightarrow$

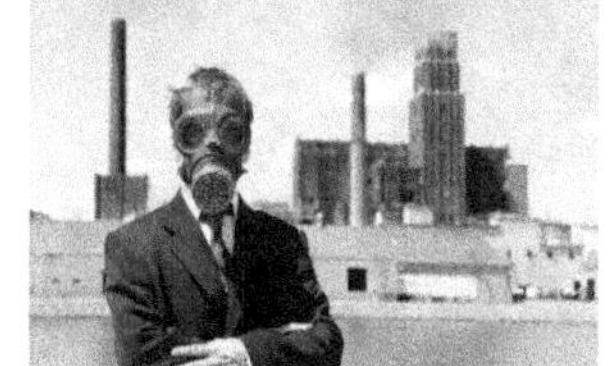

"To know that one life has breathed easier because you have lived, that is to have succeeded."

~ Ralph Waldo Emerson

b. Toxic water detoxification

Detoxify the household's water supply by purchasing a water filter. There are various kinds of filters from portable and counter top to whole house systems. In general, filters are very functional and can be easily installed on the kitchen counter or under the sink.

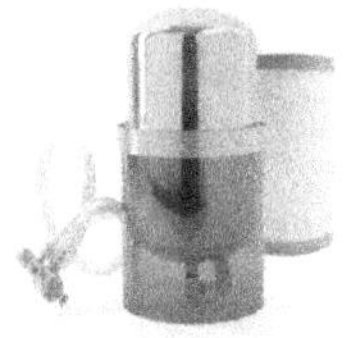

At 9 cents/gallon, this filter equals $\downarrow$

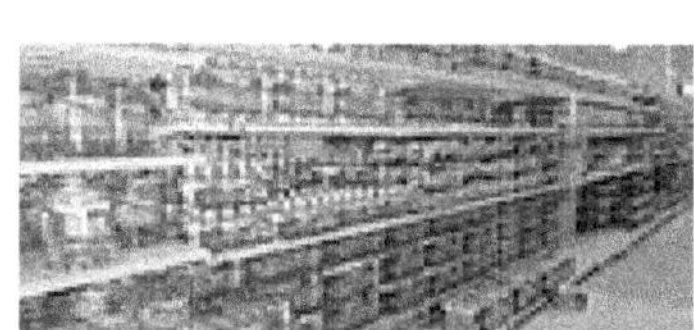

without phthalates and $\longrightarrow$

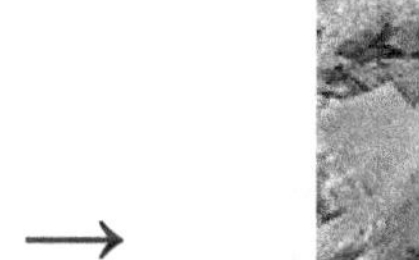

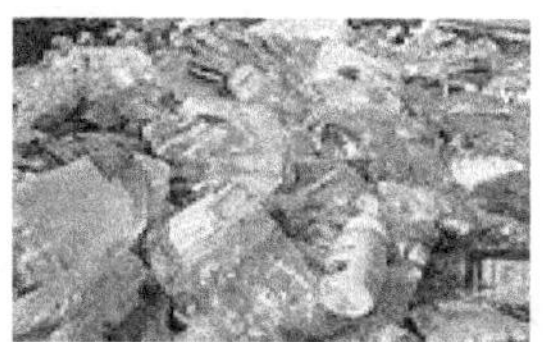

c. Kitchen cleaning and maintenance products

Take an inventory of all the cleaning products in the kitchen. Most of them are likely to be toxic. If you have not educated yourself on the matter, learn to make a distinction between toxic commercial products and green (non-toxic) products. Read product labels and proceed to identify the ingredients to know which ones are toxic.

Kitchen cleaning products come in close contact with food. Whether we wash our dishes by hands or have the dishwasher do it, there usually is a certain amount of residue left on the dishes. The cleaning products' residues are usually not quite visible but may be present on the dishes. Consequently, the residues end up being ingested with the food that comes in contact with the dish. Additionally, when we wash our dishes, if we do not have a quality water filter to get the contaminants under control, we are likely to have the contaminants from the water in contact with our food also. The quality of our meals depends not only on the quality of the meals' components but also on the quality of the detergent and water we use.

One must pay attention to words of caution and warnings on products labels. Even when there is no warning, carefully read the labels nevertheless. Some products are sometimes labeled with derivatives of names designed to hide the most popular names for toxic elements. Even some companies touting the manufacture of 'green' products often use harmful chemicals in their goods. It is self-education that encourages average consumers to become more aware and learn to detect fraudulence; when one is knowledgeable about the repercussions of the covert hazards in commercial products, it is easier to take corrective action.

d. Cookware, housewares, utilities, etc.

They have their share of hazards that must first be identified.

SOME OF THE TOXIC SUBSTANCES IN COOKWARE, HOUSEWARES, UTILITIES, MISC. CAUSES, ETC.

Types	Found in	Effects	Alternatives
Teflon - Plastic residues (they release Perfluor-inated compounds (PFCs) that are highly toxic	Non-stick cookware	Degenerative diseases	Cast iron, stainless steel, eco-friendly or 'green' utensils
Phathalates	Plastic products, beverage bottles, food containers, microwaved items containers, etc.	Degenerative diseases and endocrine disruption	Phthalates-free products
Aluminum	Cooking utensils, baking soda, foil	Alzheimer's Disease	Cast iron, stainless steel, 'green' utensils
Styrene	Plastic wraps, styrofoam, wax products	Possible cancer risk and endocrine disruption	Use wax paper or other alternatives
Phosphates	Dishwashing detergents	Immune impairment	Eco-friendly products
Radon	Water, air, (also in granite and marble but the risk is negligible)	Second cause of lung cancer after smoking	Stop smoking and seek professional radon remediation
Volatile Organic Compounds (VOCs)	Aerosol cleansing products and aerosol cooking sprays, some cleaning products	Degenerative diseases	Non aerosol products and non-toxic green products

For more benefit to the kitchen, it is necessary to do a thorough cleanse of the drain. Professional help may be required for safe cleansing, de-greasing, and disinfection.

e. Toxic food products

See the chapter on physiological detoxification

Remedies:

1. Discard all products that are known health hazards in an environmentally conscious way.

2. Explore and utilize non-toxic alternatives.

3. Be mindful of the ingredients list when shopping.

> *"The most important environmental issue is one that is rarely mentioned,*
> *and that is the lack of a conservation ethic in our culture."*
>
> ~ Gaylord Nelson

The bathroom

Many people like a sparkling clean bathroom. Often super clean bathrooms become breeding grounds for illnesses due to the high level of toxicity from the cleaning products. The fumes and VOC can linger in the air for hours and provoke symptoms of allergy and more. There are perils to be aware of when using toxic household cleaning products. Pay attention to identifying toxins when buying the next batch of bathroom products.

Bathroom products fall under two categories: products for maintenance and for personal care. Both categories contain products that present major, and sometimes fatal health hazards. To identify the hazards, know the possible causes of toxicity, take an inventory of the products, read the labels, and decide what to eliminate and what to substitute with.

Possible causes of toxicity:

1. Contaminants (dust, mold, toxic cleaning products, phthalates, etc.)

2. Stale air

3. Toxic cleaning products, toxic cookware, toxic housewares, etc.

Identification of toxins

a. Cleaning and maintenance products

Numerous manufacturers tout the benefits that make their new products more desirable than the old. The general trend for the more recently marketed products is in the direction of self-cleaning action for walls, toilet bowls, bathtubs, etc. However, the self-cleaning benefits also come with an additional load of toxic ingredients in the products. Most of these products do not have an ingredients' list but indicate in the fine print that there are health risks. Some of them are marked: 'poison' or 'flammable', or 'Harmful or fatal if swallowed'. Exercise caution when using such products in homes where there are children, particularly toddlers who are likely to explore cabinets.

SOME OF THE TOXIC SUBSTANCES IN THE BATHROOM
CLEANING AND MAINTENANCE PRODUCTS

Types	Found in	Risks	Alternatives
Chlorine	Water, detergents, scrubbing products	Degenerative diseases, allergies, lungs and sinus problems. Interferes with iodine, making one more susceptible to thyroid problems.	Use a shower filter, buy chlorine-free, eco-friendly products
Ammonia	Detergents, scrubbing products and sprays	Degenerative diseases, allergies, lungs and sinus problems	Ammonia-free, eco-friendly products
2-butoxyethanol	Bathroom cleansers	Eye, nose and throat irritation, red blood cells damage	Toxins-free cleansers
Formaldehyde (formalin)	All types of soaps and detergents	Asthma, immune system impairment, and more	Formaldehyde-free products
Volatile Organic Compounds (VOCs)	Aerosol cleaning products	Cancer and other issues	Non aerosol products and non-toxic green products
Diethanolamine (DEA) Triethanolamine (TEA)	All-purpose cleaners	Asthma and other issues	Non-toxic products
Ethylene glycol	All purpose cleansers, degreasers	Brain / nervous system damage, respiratory issues	Eco-friendly cleansers
Hydrochloric acid	Toilet bowl cleaners	Respiratory issues	Toxins-free products
Alkyl (C12-C18) benzyl-dimethylammonium chloride	Toilet bowl cleaners	Respiratory issues	Toxins-free products

Non-toxic alternative household cleaning products

Cleaning products are of great utility but are known health hazards. The three most dangerous household cleaning products are: drain cleaners, oven cleaners, and toilet bowl cleaners. It is essential to carefully read labels and be aware of the different toxic chemicals that household cleaning products contain.

In a society where deception prevails and is widely accepted as a condition to making a living, one must pay attention to words of caution and warning on products labels. Even where there is no warning, one must do due diligence by carefully reading the labels nevertheless. Remember that some products are sometimes labeled with derivatives of certain toxic ingredients' names. Remember that some companies touting the manufacture of 'green' products are using harmful chemicals in their products. It is self-education that encourages average consumers to become more aware and learn to detect fraudulence; when one is knowledgeable about the repercussions of the hazards hidden in commercial products, it is easier to take corrective action.

For personal awareness, it is useful to practice reading labels and the fine print when shopping for products. Usually when the names are unpronounceable, then they are indicative of the presence of toxic chemicals in the product.

When used in reasonable amounts and as recommended, some simple natural products can be very functional and as effective as toxic ones. Health-oriented alternatives help lessen the toxic load in the home and the environment. All of such products can easily be found at any general store. A few of them are listed in the table below:

NON-TOXIC ALTERNATIVE CLEANING PRODUCTS

Ingredients	Uses	Amount
Sodium Bicarbonate (Baking soda)	Makes an excellent scrubbing agent for sinks, tubs, counter tops, any surface that requires scrubbing	1 tsp to ½ cup, depending on size of surface to scrub
Sodium borate (Borax)	Makes an excellent scrubbing agent	1 tsp to ½ cup, depending on size of surface to scrub
Castile soap	Surface cleansing	1 tbsp in a cup of water
White vinegar	To clean windows, mirrors and glass surfaces	Dilute in water – 3 drops per quart
Lemon / lime	Surface cleansing and disinfection	As needed depending on surface
Essential oil of: lemon, cedar, or tea tree	Spray on surfaces for cleaning and disinfection	Dilute 1 to 5 drops in a quart of purified or distilled water
Hydrogen Peroxide	For bleaching and scrubbing. Is synergistically boosted by small amounts of bicarbonate.	1 tablespoon or less, depending on size of surface to clean. Dilute when necessary.

b. Personal care products

(See Chapter 11)

It is usually an interesting experience to notice how the vast majority of manufacturers of personal care products have been selling products that are known to be hazardous. Not only can the products be harmful on many levels, but also consumers tend to believe that the products are good for them.

Remedies:

1. Use alternative products and/or make your own from non-toxic ingredients.

2. Nowadays, there are alternatives to toxic products available in all green or eco-friendly stores either online or locally.

3. Contact manufacturers of toxic products and government officials to demand safer products for humans, animals, and the environment.

The basement

Possible causes of toxicity:

1. Contaminants (dust, mold, mildew, etc.)

2. Electromagnetic pollution.

3. Toxic wood from furniture materials.

4. Toxic cleaning products.

5. Stale air.

6. Pet dander.

If the basement is of the dry type, then dust and electromagnetic pollution are likely to be an issue. If it is an unfinished basement, and if there has been flooding involved, then the risk of mold and mildew is higher, in addition to the dust and electromagnetic pollution.

Remedies:

Because of health hazards that are most likely to lurk in the basement, proceed to:

1. A thorough inspection to detect hazards.

2. The removal of all toxic commercial products and replace with non-toxic ones.

3. Thoroughly dust and vacuum all surface, cleaning and polishing with non-toxic products.

4. Paying attention to get door knobs sanitized.

5. Having any and all mold and mildew professionally cleaned up and ozonated.

The laundry room

Possible causes of toxicity:

1. Hazardous chemicals (in starch spray canisters, laundry detergent, fabric softener, etc.)

2. Petrochemicals residues

3. Volatile Organic Compounds (VOCs)

Remedies:

1. Take an inventory of all items.

2. Discard what is not useful but is collecting dust.

3. Replace toxic items with non-toxic, eco-friendly ones.
    a. Heavily perfumed detergent – replace with unscented or hypoallergenic detergent.
    b. Fabric softener – replace with eco-friendly products.
    c. Use a home made fabric rinse:
    > 3 drops of cedar essential oil in the rinse water.
    > or
    > 1/3 cup of white vinegar diluted into the washing machine's water load.

The garage, shed, and other structures

Follow the same recommendations stated for the main building. Put emphasis on removing any and all hazardous petrochemical products in the places that require detoxification.

Possible causes of toxicity:

1. Dust.

2. Hazardous chemicals (insecticides, pesticides, weed killers, etc.)

3. Petrochemicals and their residues (engine oil, antifreeze, paint, kerosene, gasoline, etc.)

4. Outdated, or expired products.

5. Old car batteries.

6. All types of batteries.

Remedies:

1. Take an inventory of all items.

2. Discard what is not useful but collecting dust.

3. Properly dispose of hazardous chemicals, outdated, or expired products.

4. Contact the municipality to find out about their recycling facility and procedures to determine when and where to take certain items for eco-conscious disposal and recycling.

<u>Useful resources:</u>
1) National Institutes of Health :: Guide to household products:
   http://www.householdproducts.nlm.nih.gov
   http://www.toxnet.nlm.nih.gov
2) EPA :: Toxic cleaning products: http://www.epa.gov/kidshometour/toxic.htm
3) The Daily Green :: Phthalates: http://www.thedailygreen.com/environmental-news/latest/4885
4) Nuclear radiation protection: http://79655mi15xhk4re6l4-epp5ydm.hop.clickbank.net/
5) EPA :: A Citizen's Guide to Radon: http://www.epa.gov/radon/pubs/citguide.html
6) Environmental Working Group (EWG) :: Hall of Shame Cleaners:
http://static.ewg.org/reports/2012/cleaners_hallofshame/cleaners_hallofshame.pdf

Connecting the dots

Even though there may be no known causes for certain diseases, at least by connecting the dots between environmental toxicity and its resulting effects, we can learn to practice prevention. The number of pollutants and stressors that humans, animals, and the environment are subjected to on a daily basis is overwhelming. It is only by seeing the connection between high level toxicity and the causes of health problems that we can find workable solutions.

Cluttered mind and cluttered space

When the mind is cluttered with old unaddressed issues, toxicity, and self-doubt, there are emotional blocks preventing proper adjustment to life. The clutter in a person's home, car, and environment is a reflection of their mental clutter. What is important to know is that clutter is an unfortunate and toxic situation that leads to all sorts of health, relational, and financial problems.

> *"The things surrounding you in your home serve as subliminal reminders of who you are... Our homes will either separate us from nature or connect us to it."*
>
> ~ Denise Linn

Feng Shui as organizational strategy

In the Chinese culture, there is deep encoded wisdom. It is fascinating to see how the Chinese art of aesthetics   – also referred to as *Feng Shui* – effectively addresses the issue of clutter, disorganization and filth with perfect sense, mathematical logic, and respect for human dignity. The term Feng Shui means Wind and Water.

Feng Shui devises a logical explanation for every technique it provides as a solution to concerns regarding different aspects of our life. Whether the concerns are with our geographic location and how it affects our health or whether it is with the issues regarding the management of our emotions, Feng Shui seems to have an answer that carries the essence of timeless wisdom.

When we create a harmonious space for ourselves and our loved ones, we are less subjected to being influenced by the multiple stressors of life. It is an overload of stress that usually contributes to the development of major diseases. With the creation of new habits, we must focus on maintaining a harmonious atmosphere around us. With a non-toxic space within and outside of us, as well as a joyful disposition, we can command the resilience and dignity of the ancient sovereign Samurai.

Living in alignment with Gaia (Earth)

Lao Tzu has recommended: *"In dwelling, live close to the ground."* This recommendation makes a lot of sense considering that the closer we are to the ground, the more we are likely to benefit from the Earth's beneficial magnetic frequencies. This explains why in the old days, very sick people from the cities were sent to sanatoriums in the country to live a more natural life and often, successfully recovered. Studies have shown that the natural frequencies that emanate from the ground and travel to the bodies of the people living close to the ground have been a major factor in their recovery.

Unlike beneficial Earth frequencies, other types of energetic frequencies may adversely affect humans and animals. There are some homes with specific frequencies that can have adverse repercussions on inhabitants at the subtle energy level even though they may be totally invisible.

Additionally, on a psychological point of view, there are items in some homes that may remind the dweller(s) of events carrying a negative memory or a painful connotation. Their presence on the premises is a source of stress, therefore causes emotional toxicity. A typical stressor could be any items that remind the person of a toxic relationship, or a traumatic event in their life such as domestic violence, an accident, a tragic death, or a fire in their life. Whether they be photographs, statues, or personal items, in any case and without question, such items must be removed from the premises and disposed of. The act of disposing of such stressors can either prevent further psychological damage or assist in some form of recovery.

For levity:

"Housework can't kill you, but why take a chance?"
~ Phillis Diller

Chapter 8

Detoxification of the Business Place

*"You can't truly be considered successful in your business life
if your home life is in shambles."*

~ Zig Ziglar

There are many health hazards to be aware of in the business place. After all, the business place is what allows a working person to make a living. For many people, it is where they spend most of the day. Consequently, it is vital to ensure the ecological correctness of the work place by making sure it is properly detoxified. Just as it is the norm for home detoxification the first step toward wholeness is to remove hazards, clutter, and contaminants. In the business place, some of the contaminants are as follows:

Smoke

There was a time when people were allowed to smoke freely in the workplace. Smokers were relishing in their indulgence while violating non-smoking co-workers' right to breathe smoke-free air. Passive smoking has taken a toll on many people's health, and also taken the lives of many non-smokers. In some private offices, people still smoke indoors, just as they do in their home. Non-smokers who feel that smokers unnecessarily pollute the air in their workplace have the right to report the offense to the Occupational Safety and Health Administration (OSHA). As a government agency, OSHA is in charge of enforcing safety regulations in the workplace. http://www.osha.gov.

Volatile Organic Compounds (VOCs)

They are contaminants such as formaldehyde and xylene that are found in the air as well as in the water supply. They are by-products of petrochemicals. When water evaporates, VOCs end up

64

lingering in the air. They can also penetrate human tissues and the blood stream, contributing to health problems. Sources of VOCs in the work place usually are:

1. **Correction fluid (a.k.a. Liquid paper)**

    It contains organic solvents that are in the category of volatile organic compounds (VOCs). They are considered to be proven carcinogens and a hazard to the ozone layer. Liquid paper can be responsible for sinus and respiratory ailments, eye irritations, nausea, dizziness, and brain fog. The kind of symptoms that one may experience depends on what type of non-organic-based solvents are utilized in the product's manufacture.

    When used frequently or inhaled, White Out is a health hazard that can lead to fatalities. Some people inhale it for a cheap high. If the White Out container is tossed in the garbage and not disposed of properly, it becomes toxic to the environment.

2. Toxic fumes from cleaning products

The most common offenders are chlorine, ammonia, perfume, and other elements that give off VOCs. They can linger in the air for hours and sometimes longer. Their volatility and quick absorption are some of the reasons why they may cause health issues. Since many office buildings have neither windows nor adequate ventilation systems, they may contribute to illnesses. The way to remedy this problem is to vacate the building. If it is possible to salvage the building, one can initiate remediation in the same manner that is covered in the chapter on home detoxification. The basics of toxic fumes management are about finding safer alternatives to toxic cleaning products and ventilate.

Phthalates and Bisphenol-A

As seen in this book's chapter on environmental toxicity, phthalates and Bisphenol-A are released into water, beverages, and food by way of plastic containers. In the business place, most of the toxic contaminants related to water consumption are found in:

1) **The water cooler**

2) **Bottled water**

    a) Bottled water, in many cases, is no better than tap.
    b) In certain cases, it may be worse than tap because:
        a.a) It may develop harmful contaminants when the water becomes stagnant in the bottle.
        a.b) The phthalates and Bisphenol-A leaching out of the plastic water bottles can be vectors of degenerative diseases and endocrine disruption.

Additionally, bottled water is known to be:

1) Expensive compared to tap water.

2) Wasteful and toxic because the plastic ends up in the landfills where it eventually contaminates the waterbeds before returning to the water supply with an additional load of contaminants.

Electromagnetic Radiation (EMR)

Office machines, equipment, and related electric devices are an absolute necessity for running a business. The work place is usually equipped with different machines or devices such as computers, routers, TV sets, monitors, fax machines, copy machines, paper shredders, water coolers, microwave oven, refrigerator, telephones, smart meters, and much more. The flip side of these types of equipment is that they generate electromagnetic radiation (EMR) and the related frequencies can be hazardous.

The main sources of EMR in the work place usually are:

1. Computers

They emit electromagnetic radiation and may eventually adversely affect the DNA's structure, cause eyesight issues, fatigue, etc.

2. Cellular devices

Very much like computers do, they also emit radiation that can cause brain damage when used extensively and with direct contact to the ear.

3. All types of office machines

They also emit EMR however to a lesser extent than some computers.

4. Microwave oven

Research studies have found that microwave technology alters the molecular structure of food and water, therefore is likely to cause cell damage to the body.

Electromagnetic Frequencies (EMF)

They are mostly related to radio frequency radiation from cellular phones, BlueTooth, WiFi, iPads, smart meters, etc. Unbiased studies have shown them to pose health hazards.

Sensible detoxification solutions for the workplace

1. Make the workplace safer by getting environmental contaminants and health hazards under control.

2. If the building is under management by a third party, it is important to discuss the matter of environmental concerns with the building manager in order to reach some win-win solutions in the best interest of all.

3. Manage the electromagnetic radiation levels of the office equipment:
   . Use a Gauss meter to measure the radiation levels.
   . Disconnect the equipment if it is not in use or needed soon.
   . Invest in an EMF protection device.

4. Secure a quality water filter or at least a portable one.

5. Arrange to green the place by adding air purifying plants that do not require much sun light in order to survive or thrive.

6. Avoid using aerosol sprays.

7. Ventilate.

Useful resources:
Sources of quality water purification systems:
1. Multi Pure Corporation: 1-800-629-9206 – Distributorship #426453 – http://www.multipure.com
2. http://abetterworld.tv/water-filtration/

For levity:

Best excuses if you get caught sleeping at your work desk:

"This is just a 15-minute power nap like they raved about in the last time management course you sent me to."

"Whew! I guess I left the top off the liquid paper."

"Someone must have put decaf in the wrong pot!"

"I wasn't sleeping! I was meditating on the mission statement and envisioning a new paradigm!"

~ Anon

Chapter 9

Detoxification of the Vehicle

"We can no longer rely just on seatbelts and airbags to keep us safe in cars... Our research shows that autos are chemical reactors, releasing toxins before we even turn on the ignition. There are safer alternatives to these chemicals, and innovative companies that develop them first will likely be rewarded by consumers."

~ Jeff Gearhart,
Director of the Ecology Center's Clean Car Campaign

Where ignorance is bliss, it is folly to be wise. When it comes to advice, fools will not take it and the wise do not even need it. So, as scientists have been stating: the different grades of plastics that our cars are made of can be hazardous to our health. Some members of our population know that, but most of them choose to remain inactive when they have the opportunity to upgrade their lifestyle as it relates to the safety of their vehicle. Many people continue to spray their cars with toxic air fresheners. Some hang cardboard air freshener items on their rear view mirror. Some continue to keep plastic water bottles in the heat of the sun in their enclosed car. Others leave their windows open when they pump gasoline. Often, people who experience toxicity symptoms caused by unseen influences end up blaming their issues on the weather.

Some car owners give to their vehicle minimal care compared to what they could be doing to make their vehicle eco-friendly. If a driver is not environmentally conscious, their car is toxic. First of all, there is not much a person can do to control the different grades of chemicals that emanate from the material the vehicle is made of.

New vehicles contain toxic chemicals that affect brain function and reproductive organs. Many people seem to be addicted to the so-called new car smell. For some, it is even a status symbol. Some car maintenance products come with new car smell as a designer fragrance.

Cars contain significant amounts of phthalates that – as seen in previous chapters – are the plastic by-products that have been shown to adversely affect health because they are neurotoxins.

Hazardous chemicals can cause brain fog, headaches, confusion, and behavioral issues that may end up impairing a driver's ability to properly perform driving tasks.

If you have just acquired a new car, use the fan for at least ½ hour while the windows are open. The ventilation will allow any excess of airborne industrial by-products to be dissipated.

Solution-oriented recommendations for vehicular detoxification

Just as we have recommended for the home:
1. First unclutter. It is important to unclutter the car if it is filled with items that are not used on a regular basis. Remove every item from the car.

2. Thoroughly clean and disinfect the vehicle's interior with environmentally-friendly products.

3. Vacuum-clean to remove dust and also pay attention to vacuum-clean the ventilation ducts, dashboard, carpeting, and all crevasses.

4. Decide what items are returning inside the vehicle and clean them thoroughly. Throw away whatever else is not returning inside. The rule of thumb is: if the item has not been used in twelve months, then it is useless and is not likely to be used in the future. The exceptions to the rule would be:

    a. Car repair tools kit.
    b. Fire extinguisher.
    c. Emergency preparedness items.

5. Wash the exterior of the car.

6. Avoid air fresheners. They are likely to contain chlorofluorocarbons, limonene, phthalates, Volatile Organic Compounds (VOC), etc.

7. Use a natural cedar wood ball for the generation of pleasant odor.

Safety precautions

1. Avoid keeping plastic bottled water in the car, particularly in hot temperatures. Bottled water that has stayed in the car while exposed to extreme heat for prolonged amounts of time is likely to contain hazardous neurotoxins.

2. Use non-toxic cleaning products that are readily available in all eco-friendly stores.

3. Beware of anything marketed under the caption "All natural" because it is often an overrated buzzword. Read labels first to investigate the ingredients' list.

A recent observation of very overweight bus drivers has led to the following conclusion:

1. The driver is exposed to phthalates and other chemicals that are intrinsic to the vehicle itself for the duration of their shift, at every shift, for the duration of their assignment.

2. The driver's uniform is, in most cases, always made of synthetic materials that are likely to be hazardous to the body and mind because of the absorption of toxic chemicals.

3. The driver is likely to drink plastic-laced water and other beverages throughout the shift.

4. The driver does not have the time or the ability to access quality water and food while on the road. The type of water and food available during the driver's shift simply encourage the production of excessive body fat.

5. The driver is also exposed to enormous emissions of CO_2.

These conditions contribute to making the driver a driving toxic time bomb.

For levity:

"Road rage is the expression of the amateur sociopath in all of us, cured by running into a professional."

~ Robert Brault

Part II

PHYSIOLOGICAL TOXICITY

Chapter 10

Causes and Effects of Physiological Toxicity

"... toxic waste water, as well as accidental spills, can contaminate drinking water and harm human health."

~ David Suzuki

Physiological Toxicity

All aspects of cellular toxicity affecting the body involve physiological toxicity. All of the environmental stressors mentioned in the earlier chapters of this book contribute to toxicity.

These elements are more specifically part of the large inventory of chemical additives, preservatives, food conditioners, food colorings, emulsifiers, yeast, mold retardants, fillers, etc. that litter our food supply. This is in addition to the pesticides, herbicides, fungicides, growth hormones drugs, and other substances covered in this book's chapter on environmental toxicity. In the US only, the number of pesticides used in the food supply has been estimated at 50,000. Between 1950 and 1985, the rate of cancer increased by 32%. After the National Cancer Institute released studies evidencing an increase in incidences of cancer, the facts correlated with research indicating that additives were harmful to human health.

It takes motivation and patience to undo the pervasive mental programming that encourages toxicity and has caused people to regard a toxic life as a normal one. After correctness is established, one can engage in properly caring for the body.

"Poison is in everything and no thing is without poison.
The dosage makes it either a poison or a remedy."

~ Paracelsus

The bodies of humans and animals exhibit various physiological responses to toxic elements. Some elements are toxic, however, when introduced to the body in micro doses, they can help support bodily functions. In this case, we are referring to trace minerals, such as selenium, copper, gold, silver, magnesium, manganese, zinc, etc. Chemical additives found to be harmful must be rejected, regardless of the reason why they end up in the body.

Air toxicity
From chemical toxins to hard-to-detect microorganisms, all forms of pollutants that adversely affect the planet also affect the physiology of humans and animals. A large number of issues, from sinus problems, lungs disorder, and other issues like cancer, often exist due to polluted air supply outdoors and poor indoor air quality.

Water toxicity
Water, just like air, is vital. The quality of the mainstream water supply is questionable because of the existing pollution caused by dumping and littering. The pollutants in the air also end up in the water supply. The consumption of bottled water is not a progressive solution because of the phthalates and Bisphenol-A. These plastic by-products come in as additional pollutants with the bottles that contain commercially sold water. This type of water has also been found to contain bacteria due to the stagnation that has occurred during long-term storage.

Food toxicity
All kinds of pesticides, herbicides, fungicides, chemical fertilizers, chemical additives, food colorings, chemical food enhancers, etc., all contribute to organ dysfunction.

Personal care products toxicity
The skin is the largest organ in the body and is subjected to abusive treatment by petrochemical products and nanotechnological products that cause health problems. Most of what is applied on the skin is eventually absorbed through the pores, and over time, ends up in the blood stream, liver, kidneys and other organs.

Cleaning products toxicity
Low quality cleaning products contain chemical products that can be very toxic and hazardous to the sinus passages, the lungs, the skin, and other organs.

Microwaves toxicity
Microwaves are radio waves that comprise wavelengths measured between one millimeter and one meter, with frequencies ranging between 300 megahertz (Mh) and 300 gigahertz (Gh). Microwaving is involved in food heating, cellular communication, satellite communication, defense weaponry, etc. It affects the body at the cellular level.

Electromagnetic toxicity
Prolonged or regular exposure to electromagnetic radiation from television transmitters, cellular phones, power lines, etc. is detrimental to the body. Electromagnetic toxicity overlaps with microwave technology.

Dental care toxicity
Mercury that has been used as an ingredient in amalgam for silver-mercury dental fillings. It is very toxic and has been found to contribute to ailments such as cancer, multiple sclerosis, Parkinson's Disease, Alzheimer's Disease, to name a few.

Disease management toxicity
People with serious illness being managed with chemotherapy and radiation end up passing the by-products of such procedures through their stools, urine, and sputum into the water supply as toxins. Besides chemotherapy and radiation metabolic by-products, people's bodies also release pharmaceutical drugs residues and hormonal drugs residues into the water supply. Municipal water treatment does not yet have the technology to prevent such by-products from accessing the water from the tap.

The human body is designed to function on clean air, pure water and food, in order to experience optimum vitality and resistance to disease. With the innumerable assaults that our bodies are subjected to daily, it takes sustained strategic maintenance work to achieve even quasi-normal body functions in this day and age.

If we are to compare our personal care to the type of care that people lavish on their car, the stark contrast between the two can be shocking. Most people pay top dollars to their mechanic for regular oil change, radiator check, transmission and windshield fluid care, etc. They take their car for a car wash, turtle wax and detailing. However, the same people are in total oblivion when it comes to their personal care. Regarding anything about non-toxic nutrition or personal care, they would not know where to start. Most have never heard of self-detoxification, even once in their whole lifetime.

"What fools indeed we mortals are
To lavish care upon a car,
With ne'er a bit of time to see
About our own machinery!"

~ John Kendrick Bangs

A lot of people are walking around feeling, looking, and acting very dysfunctional. They have innumerable symptoms from skin rashes to depression or rage, from memory blanks to excessive flatulence and chronic phlegm production. They unfortunately happen to be toxic time bombs and most of their issue has to do with an out of control toxic overload. They may have serious health issues: cancer, diabetes, obesity, heart failure, kidney disease, etc. Oftentimes, their problem is mostly related to unaddressed toxicity. People's physiological toxicity dictates their decreased quality of life. Symptoms are like red lights on a vehicle's dashboard: they indicate that an issue needs to be urgently handled. Ignoring or suppressing symptoms equates covering up a dashboard's red light warning a driver that the car is low on motor oil.

The food supply: what to detoxify from

The American food supply has been found to contain over 10,000 chemicals, many of them are banned in Europe. The chemicals are in the food not because of health requirements but out of industrial ingenuity and creativity regarding a need to maximize profit. Below is an overview of some of the most blatant toxic substances that are present in the food supply.

SOME OF THE TOXIC ELEMENTS IN THE FOOD SUPPLY

Types	Found in	Effects	Alternatives
Pesticides	Non-organic produce, foreign and GMO produce	Degenerative diseases	Natural fertilizers
Herbicides	Non-organic produce, foreign and GMO produce	Alzheimer's disease	Detoxify

Heavy metals:
    aluminum
    mercury
    arsenic
    lead
    cadmium
    boron
	Soda cans, deodorant, baking supplies
	High fructose corn syrup (HFCS)
	Chicken
	Water
	Water
	Water
		Heavy metals toxicity	Detoxify

Food preservatives	All commercially packaged foods and beverages	Endocrine dysfunctions, low testosterone count	Detoxify
Food additives	All commercially packaged foods and beverages	Endocrine dysfunctions, low testosterone count	Detoxify
Food conditioners	Commercially prepared food and beverages	DNA damage / weight issues other health issues	Detoxify
Food dyes (FD&C)	Countless commercial foods, chewing gum	DNA damage / weight issues other health issues	Detoxify and avoid FD&Cs
Yeast	Bread and bread / wheat products	Candida albicans, nail fungus, behavioral issues, allergies, etc.	Yeast free products
Bisphenol -A / Phthalates	Water, plastics, packaging, canned food	Cancer risk, endocrine issues	Detoxify
Nitrates / Nitrites	Bacon, cold cuts, preserved foods	Cancer risk, allergies	Detoxify
Biotech / GMO hazards	Most non-organic food	Risk of DNA damage	Detoxify / buy organic grow your own food
Food irradiation	Meats, herbs, spices, etc.	DNA damage	Detoxify
Processed sugar	Many types of food	Dental cavities, behavioral issues, immune suppression, parasitic infestation	Honey, xylitol
Monosodium Glutamate (MSG)	Commercial foods, oriental food	Excessive weight gain, obesity, diabetes, organs dysfunction, macular degeneration, etc.	Avoid MSG
Trans fats	Commercial foods, fried foods	Mitochondria damage, obesity, overweight conditions, etc.	Avoid trans fats
Parasites	Milk, pork, sushi, water, unclean hands, blood, excrement, clothing, bedding, shoes, etc.	Travel from one host to another cause a multitude of symptoms	Practice cleanliness, avoid sugar and excess meat
Antibiotics residues	Frozen fish, meats from animals treated with antibiotics	Drug resistance	Avoid frozen fish and buy free-range meats
Growth hormones	Beef, chicken, etc.	Excessive estrogen	Grain-fed or free range

Facts about the food supply

Not all types of food are equal. There are some major differences between natural and processed foodstuff when it comes to nutritional value.

Because people can be oblivious to the interaction between food as nourishing agent and its direct influence on bodily functions, they often become accustomed to eating what is convenient, rather than what is necessary for normal sustenance. Unfortunately, when people stay on deficient diets for prolonged amounts of time, they develop physical problems in the form of: obesity, extra fat production, osteoporosis, cognitive dysfunction, sleep problems, to name a few.

. Home grown food has a higher nutritional value than processed food and biotech food.
. Home-cooked food has a higher nutritional value than industrially prepared food.

Cattle is injected with: bovine growth hormones, antibiotics, tranquilizers, etc.

Fruits and vegetables are sprayed with pesticides to prevent insects from devouring them before harvest. They are also treated with fungicides to retard mold attacks.

The following contains the Environmental Working Group's most recent list of the most sprayed vegetables and fruits and a list for the least sprayed produce.

Most sprayed:	Least sprayed:
Apples	Asparagus
Strawberries	Avocado
Grapes	Cabbage
Celery	Cantaloupe
Cucumbers	Sweet corn
Cherry tomatoes	Eggplant
Hot peppers	Grapefruit
Bell peppers	Kiwi
Spinach	Mango
Nectarines (imported)	Mushrooms
Peaches	Onions
Summer squash	Papaya
Kale	Pineapple
Collard greens	Sweet peas (frozen)
Potatoes	Sweet potatoes

Useful resources:
1. The Doctor's TV: http://www.thedoctorstv.com/main/show_synopsis_print/779
2. GMO: http://grist.org/article/gmo-fail-monsanto-foiled-by-bedg-supreme-court-and-science/
3. GMO: http://www.amazon.com/gp/product/B007X8NH34?ie=UTF8&seller=A1D0QAQWKX0LCW&sn=ABetterWorld

Food has different grades of bio-availability depending on its source and the way it has been processed. In general:

Naturally grown food is a lot more nutritive than processed food.

Raw or minimally cooked or minimally processed food is higher in nutritional value than:
        •commercially-prepared or processed food
        •frozen food
        •canned food
        •stewed food
        •microwaved food
        •charcoal- cooked food

Food packaged in plastic has a higher level of phthalates and Bisphenol-A than food stored in glass or ceramic.

The processing of food is intended to keep it from spoiling before it reaches the food store shelf. It involves preventing insects from destroying the food in the fields; it also involves genetic engineering to make the food less attractive to insects and more resistant to impact during transportation which often involves coast to coast travel and importation from overseas.

Some processed food is manufactured to last for years without refrigeration. This type of food can come very handy in cases of natural disasters but is not to be consumed on a regular basis.

In general, the processing of food also entails rendering the food non bio-active in the case of fruits of vegetables. This simply means that the food has to be killed so that it can be preserved indefinitely. Long- term use of this type of foodstuff usually leads to bodily imbalances because it is devoid of the life force and nutrients that replenish life. It is life that replenishes life.

Many people systematically avoid eating fruits or vegetables because they are more accustomed to processed food. They neither understand nor trust the process of life to sustain them. In fact, they may even ask if eating certain fruits or vegetables is harmful to them! In the homes of the most toxic people, there may not be any fruits and vegetables. In the rare events that produce may be brought in, it is likely to sit around, ignored for weeks, while rotting. Very toxic people mostly purchase fast food, fried and processed meats, sugar, soft white bread, alcohol, and soda as regular staple.

"We are living in a world today where lemonade is made from artificial flavors and
furniture polish is made from real lemons."

~ Alfred E. Newman

Personal care products and other items: what to detoxify from

Most personal care products are *weaponized*. Even brands touting natural ingredients also market toxic products.

Some of the most toxic products are those marketed for baby care. They often contain neurotoxins that are disruptive to the lymphatic, hormonal, and endocrinological systems.

SOME OF THE TOXIC SUBSTANCES IN PERSONAL CARE PRODUCTS

Types	Found in	Risks	Alternatives
Sodium lauryl sulfate, Sodium laurel sulfate, Sodium laureth sulfate, Sodium myreth sulfate	Shampoo, liquid soap, bath soap, etc.	Degenerative diseases, hair loss	SLS-free products
Formaldehyde (released by Quaternium-15, 2-bromo-2- nitropropane-1, 3-diol, DMDM hydantoin, imidazolidinyl urea, etc.)	Baby and adult bath liquid soaps, shampoos, hair conditioners, creams and lotions, hair care and hair grooming products, skin remedies products, etc.	Health issues such as cancer and immune system impairment	Formaldehyde-free products
Propylene Glycol	Mouthwash, creams, lotions, shampoos, conditioners, shaving cream, hair spray, gels, deodorant, grooming products, spermicides, personal lubricants, vaginal creams, etc.	Cancer and other health issues	Toxins-free products
Parabens	Creams, lotions, conditioners, and more	Cancer and other health issues	Toxins-free products
Carbomer	Creams, lotions and many more skin care products	Cancer and other health issues	Toxins-free products
PEG	Creams, lotions and many more skin care products	Degenerative diseases	Toxins-free products
Ceteareth, oleth, etc.	Creams, lotions and many more skin care products	Degenerative diseases	Toxins-free products
Lye	Hair straighteners	Degenerative diseases, hair loss, etc.	Plant–based relaxers
Fragrances (artificial)	Most personal care products	Allergies, lung issues, phthalates-related issues	Fragrance-free products
Xynol	Cosmetics and cleaning products	Respiratory issues and other health problems	Toxins-free products
Triclosan	Antibacterial soaps, deodorants, etc.	Rashes, kidney damage acid mantle damage	Toxins-free products
Acetone	Nail polish remover	Cancer and lung issues	Acetone-free products

Basically, the rule of thumb is: if the product has a warning on its label, *caveat emptor* (Latin term for: "Let the buyer beware"). For instance, all mainstream toothpastes carry on their label a warning that comes in a very fine print as:

> **Warnings:** Keep out of the reach of children under 6 years of age. If more than used for brushing is accidentally swallowed, get medical help or contact a Poison Control Center right away.

Useful resources:
1. http://downwithbasics.com/the-5-hidden-dangers-in-toothpaste
2. http://www.mercola.com/Downloads/bonus/toxic-personal-care-products/report.aspx
3. http://www.drfranklipman.com/personal-care-products-pose-unrecognized-toxic-risks-to-children/
4. http://www.toxnet.nlm.nih.gov
5. http://www.scorecard.org
6. http://www.atsdr.cdc.gov/toxfaqs/ft.asp?id=4&tid=1

Some toxins in personal care products and cosmetics have also been found to cause:
- brain fog
- cognitive issues
- vision problems including blindness

Often overlooked toxic stressors: parasites

The existence of parasites in the human body is an ecological fact. When food stagnates in the intestines, parasites proliferate and oftentimes because pathogenic.

Foodsafety.gov defines parasites as follows:
"Parasites are organisms that derive nourishment and protection from other living organisms known as hosts. Many of these organisms can be transmitted by water, soil, or person-to-person contact. Parasites range in size from tiny, single-celled organisms to worms visible to the naked eye. In the United States, the most common foodborne parasites are protozoa, roundworms, and tapeworms. The foodborne parasite that causes the most hospitalizations and deaths in this country is Toxoplasma gondii, which causes toxoplasmosis." http://www.foodsafety.gov/poisoning/causes/parasites/index.html

Everyone, to a certain degree – especially meat and produce eaters – is a host to parasites, internally and/or externally. Constipated people have more parasites than others, so do people who do not care to sanitize their hands. Parasites are easily transmissible through handshakes, touching, feeding, sexual activity, drinking unclean water, using unclean clothes and bedding, to say the least. Dr. Shuktan attests to these facts on Dr. Oz's show as can be seen on the video in this link: http://www.youtube.com/watch?v=yRglUAttmzQ

Parasites are usually very small in size, some of them microscopic. They thrive in water, the soil, foods (deteriorating food and raw food such as sushi), produce, blood, the bowels, excrement, internal organs, and also thrive on unkempt humans, household pets, birds, and soiled items. They are highly intelligent and are designed to survive in the harshest environment.

Parasites thrive in water, on produce, and particularly, in the bodies of humans and animals. Organic produce can be host to parasites more than non-organic produce that has been treated with pest control chemicals.

Parasites are also known to mind-control their host. This phenomenon is explained in this video: http://www.livescience.com/7019-mind-control-parasites.html

People who are subjected to frequent foods cravings particularly foods that are high in processed sugar, may be under parasitic control. One of the easiest way to contract parasites is by eating pork. Even when pork is fried at very high temperatures, it may harbor plenty of seemingly indestructible parasites.

Due to age-old indoctrination and propaganda, most people believe that in so-called developed countries, the majority of the people is exempt from parasitism because they are oblivious to the existence of parasites. Usually, the subject of parasites is carefully avoided because not only it is embarrassing to discuss, but also it is not politically correct. Not only ignorance is bliss, but also, people have a tendency to deny what they fear or think is too gross to handle.

In cities with a large population density, some the most parasites-infested surfaces are: door knobs, highly trafficked public areas, money changing hands often, and public vehicles. Many people have been contaminated by lice just by having their head in contact with the seats of infested public vehicles.

Some symptoms of parasitism:
    . Chronic fatigue
    . Irritability
    . Mood swings
    . Cravings
    . Frequent hunger
    . Inability to feel full even after a large meal
    . Weight gain
    . Obesity
    . Drooling
    . Diarrhea
    . Itching (skin, anus)

Parasites are a most carefully avoided subject but their presence in the body contributes to health and behavioral issues. For the issue to be properly addressed, one must first know the enemy.

SOME OF THE PARASITES CONTRIBUTING TO TOXICITY

Types	Found where?	Effects	Action to take
INTERNAL:			
Giardia	Unclean water	Diarrhea	Seek medical help, detox
Ascaris (giant round worm)	Human intestines, unclean places	Weakness, diarrhea, growth retardation, etc. flu symptoms, anal itch	Seek medical help, detox
Tapeworm	Human intestines, beef or pork, dogs, cats	Anal itch, abdominal discomfort	Seek medical help, detox
Toxoplasmosis	Human tissues	Pain, fatigue, seizures, swollen lymph nodes, fever	Seek medical help, detox
EXTERNAL:			
. Lice	Human heads, pets	Rashes, itching	Seek medical and exterminator help
. Mites	Dust, unclean surfaces, dogs' ears	Allergies and more	Thorough clean living quarters
. Bed bugs	Anywhere, even in clean places, hotels	Severe rashes, allergies	Seek professional exterminator help
. Some species of fungi	Dark, moist places, nails, skin, hair	Destruction of nails, skin, and hair follicles	Seek medical help, detox
. Ringworm (more of a fungus than a worm)	Skin, nails, scalp, beard, groin, etc.	Redness, itchy rash	Seek medical help, detox

In some obese people, one-third of their intestinal contents is loaded with fecal matter produced by the parasites that inhabit their body.

Useful resources:

1. USDA Food Safety and Inspection Service:
http://www.fsis.usda.gov/FACTSheets/Parasites_and_Foodborne_Illness/index.asp
2. Discover Magazine – Tapeworms in the brain:
http://discovermagazine.com/2012/jun/03-hidden-epidemic-tapeworms-in-the-brain

Resistance to hygiene contributes to toxicity

Statistics gathered from a study by the American Society of Microbiology have shown that only 50 percent of men wash their hands after using the toilet compared to 75 percent of women. Middle and high school students observed throughout the study led the conclusion that only 8 percent of males washed their hands as opposed to 33 percent of females.

On an individual level, one can greatly contribute to minimizing the spread of illnesses caused by parasites, harmful pathogen, simply by washing one's hands conscientiously and avoiding direct contact with public door surfaces, particularly door knobs. A research conducted in London speculated that if everyone were to routinely wash their hands, one million lives would be saved from contagious illnesses each year.

It is puzzling to see how some people eat bananas. Though bananas come with a perfect, easy peel-off design that makes it easy to eat the fruit without touching its pulp, many people peel bananas off, throw away the peel then hold the unpeeled banana to eat it, without washing either their hands or the fruit beforehand. This habit may contribute to the introduction of pesticides and disease-causing germs into the banana's pulp.

There was a health-oriented man of goodwill, an educator, a mover-and-shaker from a metropolis, who traveled to suburbia to pay a benevolent visit to a lady friend. Upon arriving in suburbia, the good man mentioned how complex and time-consuming it was for him to leave his high-rise apartment, ride his vehicle to the nearest subway station, park his vehicle nearby, take a subway ride to the bus, then ride the bus to his friend's suburban apartment building. His hostess offered him a meal and showed him where the bathroom was. When the guest began partaking of the meal without making a move to go wash his hands, the hostess asked him whether he would want to go sanitize his hands before eating. The guest replied: "Oh, no thank you. I didn't touch anything." The hostess then asked him whether he had closed his apartment door securely, pushed an elevator button to transport himself to the ground floor, maneuvered his vehicle's steering wheel, touched the money he used to pay for his subway tokens, turned the subway trestle, touched money to pay his bus fare, pushed the elevator buttons to eventually reach the hostess' apartment. The man acknowledged doing all that. The hostess then said: "*I wonder how you got to do all that without 'touching anything'.*"

Hand sanitizers are great conveniences to have in case water and soap are not available. They are however, not a substitute for conscientious hand washing with soap and water. They are not designed for long-term or daily use but. Sanitizers do kill germs, but their repeated use may also damage the skin's acid mantle. Overuse of hand sanitizers contributes to resistance to germs. Hand sanitizers have also been found to contain substances that are known endocrine disruptors.

Toxins in clothing

There was a time when clothing was made of some of the most known natural fibers: cotton, linen, wool, and silk. With the advent of pesticides and the industrial revolution, clothing is now -- just like food, water, air, personal care products and anything else -- *weaponized*. Pesticides are sprayed on cotton and other materials that clothing is made of. Besides pesticides, there are other products that enter into the manufacture of clothing. All such products are likely to pose a cancer-causing risk and facilitate endocrine disruption. Nowadays, a lot of the world's available clothing is manufactured with synthetic chemicals like polyester, rayon, viscose, spandex, etc. Some well-known toxins, including Teflon, are now routinely used in the manufacture of clothing and accessories. Even a lot of health-oriented gym goers have no idea that their clothing is toxic. This is very much the same blind spot that many people have about sports drinks. Wearing toxic clothing is the equivalent of wearing a toxic polyester patch all over the body: it allow the toxins to penetrated the body through the pores.

Greenpeace has been reporting the sad fact that the fashion industry has been mass-marketing clothing contaminated with hazardous chemicals known to harm the immune system, therefore causing cancer, and also known to damage the endocrine system. Yifang Li, senior toxics campaigner at Greenpeace East Asia has been quoted as saying: *"Major fashion brands are turning us all into fashion victims by selling us clothes that contain hazardous chemicals that contribute to toxic water pollution around the world, both when they are made and washed."*
http://ens-newswire.com/2012/11/20/greenpeace-exposes-toxic-chemicals-in-fashionable-clothing/

Toxic products are routinely and mindlessly utilized in clothing and its finishing process. Some of these toxic products are used to maintain a shiny or permanently creased look. Countless people who wish to look sharp wear such clothing, unaware of the toxic health hazards.

From the toxins found in the production and finishing of clothing to the toxins acquired during washing, drying, and laundering, everyone is exposed to toxicity.

Useful resources:
http://grist.org/list/2011-08-23-do-your-clothes-contain-toxic-chemicals/
http://ens-newswire.com/2012/11/20/greenpeace-exposes-toxic-chemicals-in-fashionable-clothing/
http://total-health-magazine.com/articles/allergies-asthma/consumers-beware-toxins-lurking-in-your-clothing.html

Toxins in laundry products

Studies of laundry products have revealed that there are some nanotechnological hazards in such products and they can adversely affect human health. The term *nano* refers to any particle that is less than 1 micron in size. The particle happens to be so small that it is microscopic, therefore capable of penetrating the body through the pores. Because clothing is in direct contact with the skin for prolonged period of time, there is a fair amount of absorption that takes place. The quality of the laundry products one uses directly impacts the skin, the largest organ in the body.

Useful resources:
http://www.centerforfoodsafety.org/wp-content/uploads/2012/07/NANO-EXPOSED_FINAL.pdf
http://www.debralynndadd.com/Default.aspx?SiteSearchID=3284&ID=/search&Collections=X&OT=7,6

Toxins in footwear and accessories

Who has not worn plastic or latex shoes that are so convenient on the beach, or in the shower at the gym or spa? People have been wearing them in an effort to shield their feet from sharp objects and contaminants from other people who may have athlete's foot or toe nails fungus.

The footwear industry has been utilizing toxic materials in the production of their goods. Even leather shoes have been found to be laced with dangerous chemicals. Just like clothing is weaponized, footwear and accessories may carry undesirable toxins such as phthalates. Thanks to Greenpeace, the word is now out that high-end footwear manufacturers, such as Nike, Puma, and Adidas are committing to remove toxins from their manufacturing process.

Useful resources:
http://ezinearticles.com/?Toxic-Shoes&id=4371015
http://all4women.co.za/health-and-wellness/health-articles/toxins-shoes.html
http://www.gbb.org/news/wearing-toxins-how-nike-puma-and-adidas-are-removing-toxins-from-their-manufacturing-process/

Lifestyle-related toxic stressors

They usually make the body more acidic than it needs to be and are known to cause degenerative diseases as well as chemical imbalances.

Toxic environmental stressors

Among the numerous other stressors that exist, some of them are: airborne micro-organisms, free radicals (they adversely affect humans because of their toxicity, free-radical damage occurs within the mitochondria), vaccines, microwaving, EMRs, EMFs, etc.

An article published by Amanda Leigh Mascarelli published in *Medicus* from Case Western Reserve University School of Medicine clarifies the issue of pathogens:
http://www.case.edu/medicus/magazine/winter202/feature/microbes-vs-mankind.html

SOME UNSEEN AND UNACCOUNTED TOXIC STRESSORS

"A great deal of intelligence can be invested in ignorance."

~ Saul Bellow

Toxic stressors considered probable, unproven, or unknown

Some people agree that vaccines, microwave ovens, fluoride, and EMFs from cell phones are harmful. Some others disagree. Many studies tend to reflect the views and desires of the industries that promote them. Everyone is urged to do their own research and see what works best for them. Experience brings about the highest level of knowledge. There are tools and methods of measurement that help humans determine what is either beneficial or detrimental to them. Some gauging methods include Gauss meters, Hz frequency meters, and kinesiology tests.

SOME OTHER PROBABLE STRESSORS CONSIDERED UNKNOWN, UNSEEN, OR UNPROVEN		
Types	**Features**	**For protection**
Vaccines	Mercury, aluminum, formaldehyde, thimerosal, antigen, live viruses, bacterial toxins, bacterial polysaccharides, preservatives such as MSG, etc.	Detoxify.
Microwaving	Oscillating electromagnetic waves (radio-like waves)	Detoxify.
Fluoride	Water, toothpaste	Detoxify, use water filter.
Cell phones, computers, TV radiation, EMRs, EMFs, etc.	Possible DNA damage from cell phones, electronic devices, etc.	Detoxify, wear protective devices.

When it comes to hazards and unproven technologies, buyer beware. We also have to be aware that each industry has its apologists and lobbyists who influence the public's perception and acceptance of their products. Usually, big corporate interests with the most money, the most enforcement power, the loudest voice, the biggest stick or the largest carrot command the most public obedience and compliance. While the disagreement's toll is mounting in the name of science, so is the rate of toxicity-related diseases in the whole world. It appears that for sincere people, a sensible approach to an answer is to do their own research, due diligence, and seek inner wisdom, including ancient indigenous wisdom.

> *"All truth passes through three stages. First, it is ridiculed. Second, it is violently opposed. Third, it is accepted as being self-evident"*

~ Arthur Schopenhauer, German philosopher (1788 – 1860)

Useful resources:
1) Dr. Leonard Coldwell :: Microwave ovens: http://www.youtube.com/watch?feature=endscreen&NR=1&v=ScbbQ2pYd9I
2) The FDA :: Microwaving:
   http://www.fda.gov/Radiation-EmittingProducts/ResourcesforYouRadiationEmittingProducts/ucm252762.htm
   http://www.sdbest.com/Food_Safety/microwave.html
3) Products for radiation pollution control: http://abetterworld.tv/wellness/health-and-healing/energetic-balancing/

Donald Lines Jacobus drives an enlightening point in explaining that there are no exact sciences and his wisdom can serve well until there are science-based foolproof systems: *"Science" is merely a word of Latin derivation meaning "knowledge." If we except mathematics, which is not so much a science in itself as a mode of measurement employed in all the sciences, there are no exact sciences. The more definitely measurement can be employed, the more exact a science becomes. Hence, astronomy and physics may be considered as reasonably exact sciences, though even here when we approach infinite magnitude, as of distance in astronomy, or infinite smallness, as of electrons in physics, and our measuring devices are not sufficiently acute, we discover a wide margin of inexactitude.*

Sciences which relate wholly or in part to human nature are considered the least exact.

Authoritative monopolies do an impressive job solving human problems through the use of technologies that are considered to be marvels of scientific advances. They function with strong emphasis on logical, scientific, and speedy processes that respond well to the average population's needs. There are people whose needs are a lot more complex and whose understanding of technological manipulation is a lot more sophisticated than that of the majority of the populace. When it comes to making a difference in paradigms, it seems that what counts is a good understanding of causality and a far-sighted concern with end results rather than temporary fixes. There are other people whose mission is to utilize technologies that only are in humanity's best interest. For the longest time, indigenous people have often been regarded as primitive, naïve, or ignorant because they are different. Even though, they did not have access to technologically advanced processes or weaponry, indigenes have demonstrated functional wisdom. For the most part, indigenous wisdom has been more constructive than destructive to the planet. It has mostly been based on respect for human life and reverence for the environment.

Until advanced sciences bring a solid solution to the complex issues of human disease and helplessness, we are to rely on the timeless wisdom of the body to find relief. If we are only focusing on the 1% that we think we know or what we believe indigenes do not know, how then can we find out about the 99% that are not even aware that we do not know?

For levity:

A woman asked her husband to go pick up some organic vegetables for that night's dinner on his way home. At the store, the husband searched all over for organic vegetables before finally asking the produce clerk where they might be. The produce clerk said he didn't know what he was talking about, so the husband said: "These vegetables are for my wife. Have they been sprayed with poisonous chemicals?" The produce clerk replied, "No, sir, you will have to do that yourself."

~ Anon

Chapter 11

Obesity and Excess Body Fat

"We don't need new discoveries or new inventions to reverse this trend. We have the tools at our disposal to reverse it. All we need is the motivation, the opportunity and the willpower to do what needs to be done..."

~ First Lady Michelle Obama on obesity

The Times of India has recently reported in an article entitled *Obesity in 20s Cuts Chances of A Long Life*: "Every unit increase in body mass index (BMI) corresponds to an increased heart attack rate of 5 per cent, high blood pressure and blood clot rates of 10 per cent, and a raised diabetes rate of 20 per cent."

Source: http://articles.timesofindia.indiatimes.com/2013-04-30/health/38929622_1_clot-middle-age-heart-attack

In pre-industrial ages, recorded history has not reported such a thing as the epidemiological rate of obesity, excessive body weight, cancer, diabetes, and more; numerous other conditions are now being experienced in alarming proportions on the planet.

Researchers agree that the main factors involved in the issues of obesity and excess body fat are:

1. Toxicity overload from:
   - Environmental stressors.
   - Food toxicity (from artificial ingredients some of which are artificial sugar such as high fructose corn syrup in foodstuff known as pancake syrup, sodas, etc.)
   - Free radicals from fried foods.
   - Microbiological predators such as parasites, yeast organisms, etc.
   - Chronic dehydration.
   - A sedentary lifestyle.

2. Nutritional deficiencies from:
   - Low quality nutritionally deficient, empty calorie type of fatty foodstuff.
   - Poor eating habits, reckless eating schedule, meals skipping, etc.

Fat cells are toxic cells

There are people who are so toxic that their body has to constantly produce extra fat to protect them from attacking their major organs. This is one of the reasons why some people cannot lose weight easily, in spite of dieting. At times, many people who engage in dieting experience a yo-yo effect: they diet for a while and end up gaining the weight back with 'interest'. After losing ten pounds or so, they end up gaining back fifteen more pounds within two to three weeks.

A lot of consumers are not aware that there are growth hormones in meat, mostly beef and chicken. In the cattle industry, growth hormones are routinely injected in animals for fast growth and higher than normal fatty meat production. For instance, growth hormones cause a baby calf to mutate into a full-grown cow within just a few weeks, a process which would normally take several months. Since we are what we eat, when we eat hormone-laced meats, our body is more likely to metabolize the hormones the same way the animals we ate did. Eventually, the resulting effect is that the body starts producing flabby muscles and more fat.

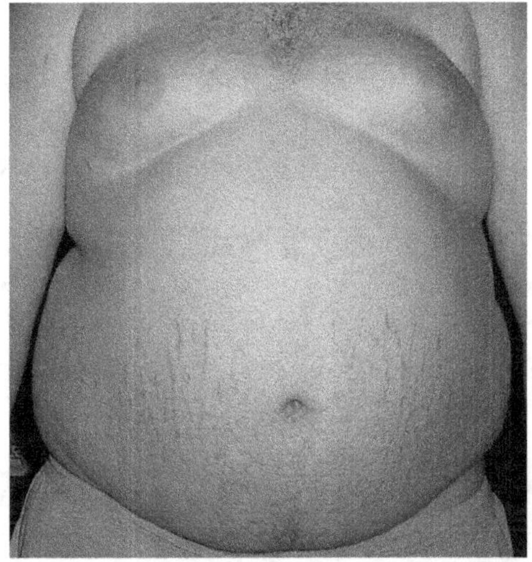

Source: commons.wikimedia.org

Overweight and obese people: overfed but malnourished

The human physiology requires that we eat a sensible diet that is to include water, fats, carbohydrates, vitamins, minerals, and protein. All these essentials are found in foods, in various degrees depending on the quality of the food.

In a society where the concept of food is blurred to the point where people believe that lunch meat, processed cheese, jelly donuts, and sodas are suitable for human consumption, it is important to make the distinction that foodstuff (junk food) is not food. Processed cheese, for instance, is said to be one molecule away from... plastic. It is more or less the same kind of plastic that releases dangerous levels of Bisphenol-A and phthalates which cause endocrine issues, cancer, and more. In this day and age, foodstuff is used as a weapon of self-destruction and ends up working as well for mass destruction.

Prolonged or excessive consumption of foodstuff causes people to experience deficiencies because the foodstuff has none of the nutrients that the body requires to function properly. Foodstuff has high caloric value that would be helpful if the consumer were to require protection from sub-zero degree temperatures. Unless one lives in the North Pole or works in a profession demanding arduous physical exertion high caloric food is hazardous to health. Most foodstuff is loaded with processed sugar and trans fats. Processed sugar robs the body of whatever reserves of nutrients it may have left. That is why people on regular foodstuff have uncontrollable and frequent hunger. In addition to that, parasites may easily take over. Trans fats are notorious for contributing to cardio vascular diseases. They are known to cause arterial blockage and may lead to a heart attack. Due to nutritional deficiencies and potential parasitic infestation, the foodstuff consumer is always hungry and looking for more junk to consume. Parasites living in the body love junk food and sugar. Because parasites can control their host's mind, the host is always looking to eat increasingly larger amounts of fatty, sugar-filled junk. Soon enough, the resulting effect is: distended stomach and abdomen, excessive fat on the body, flabbiness (e.g. jelly belly and muffin tops), fatigue, lethargy, depression, irritability, over-acidity, body odor, poor circulation, skin problems, hypertension, diabetes, cancer, etc.

Because of the lethargy that usually accompanies the consumption of foodstuff, the consumer of foodstuff seems to have a predilection for lying on a couch or bed to replenish their energy for hours at a time. This activity -- or lack of action that is -- causes the person to incur very poor digestion because food does not get normally digested during slumber or prolonged inaction.

For the body to function at optimal efficiency, it requires sensible detoxification plus a substantial quantity of nourishing nutrients that eventually get processed by the bodily organs for the maintenance of adequate function. The problem with getting adequate levels of daily nourishment is the quality of food we ingest. It is not easy to get quality from the mainstream food supply. Due to soil depletion, over farming, chemical pesticides and herbicides overuse, genetic modification, whatever food we may access is likely to be mostly devoid of the nutrients we require for optimal health. Processed food generally has been found to have a nutritional value of 20% or much less compared to non- processed, adequately grown food. Nutritionists recommend that people learn to properly supplement with nutrients that are of the adequate frequency range for initiating revitalization.

Starvation diets cause toxicity

In very toxic individuals, the fat production can be out of control; such people may gain weight simply by eating salad greens. There are many dieters who have tried to skip meals or stop eating. This type of self-treatment is abusive; it can cause other problems to the body in addition to excessive weight gain. Toxic people who skip meals are those who have the hardest time reducing their weight because when in starvation mode, the body systematically stores more fat. Those who starve themselves for a while are the ones who usually see their appetite go on a rebound and come back with a vengeance by incurring binge eating. The body has its own wisdom and coping strategies: if it interprets your starvation diet as an intention to terminate its program, it will go into challenge mode and prepare itself for combat and ultimate survival. The body prepares itself for survival by storing fat and getting it from wherever it can. The fat storage process also includes producing much more cholesterol than normally required. Starvation diets and the habit of skipping meals may also cause cravings and excessive hunger during times of major stress. When the cravings manifest, they are never for healthy foods, but for the high caloric, fattiest foodstuff. This happens because the body is under stress and is looking to produce more fat and more cholesterol to protect itself from death.

Long-term toxicity may manifest itself in the form of chronic diseases. When one feeds the body material that is not conducive to detoxifying and replenishing, disease sets in. It is very much the equivalent of running a pricy car on diesel and expect it to perform like a race car running on high octane fuel.

Diet sodas cause weight gain

Sodas are toxic and fattening; diet sodas are even worse. The majority of people who consume diet sodas and sugar-free products are brainwashed into believing that just because a product is marked 'diet' or 'sugar-free', then it can be slimming. In reality, because of the artificial sugar's detriment to the body, the surest way to get fat and obese is by consuming diet sodas and sugar-free drinks. They have major disadvantages such as:

- Tricking the body into preparing itself to ingest more food than needed.
- Causing excessive cravings, frequent hunger, and a demand for more soda (more sugar).
- Changing metabolism and brain chemistry.
- Causing a pH imbalance and acidifying the body, therefore inviting disease.
- Causing osteoporosis due to an imbalance in the phosphorus to calcium ratio.
- Encouraging kidney disease: http://www.webmd.com/diet/news/20091102/diet-sodas-hard-on-the-kidneys

The Reader's Digest has published the results of a research study on diet sodas as follows:
"Data from this and other prospective studies suggest that the promotion of diet sodas and artificial sweeteners as healthy alternatives may be ill-advised," said study researcher Helen P. Hazuda, professor at the University of Texas's school of medicine. *"They may be free of calories, but not of consequences."*

The role of opioids in overeating

Opioids are psychoactive chemicals found either in controlled substances, narcotics, and toxic foods. They can also be produced in a toxic body where they are found mainly in the nervous system and the gastrointestinal system. Opioids produce a feel-good effect when one smells or eats certain foods. In each system, there are receptors that negotiate the feel-good effects as well as the withdrawal symptoms that are related to the production of opioids. There is noted interconnectedness between food ingestion and the effects of opioids which, in general, encourage the body to desire more wheat, sugar, and fatty foods. Opioids cause an artificial 'high'. When certain toxic foods are ingested, just as it is for narcotics, a person requires more and more opioid-producing foods to maintain a certain level of satisfaction. Highly processed refined sugar shocks the body due to its high caloric intake plus then ensuing negative nutrition, both of which lead to nutrient deficiencies. Junky toxic food has significant opioid-like effects, which explains why junk food is so addictive. These facts also help understand why it is so hard for people to stay off junk food when they are very toxic and used to it for a long time. Because of these issues, toxic people who are overweight and obese require as much detoxification and rehabilitation as those addicted to drugs and alcohol. When brain chemistry issues account for opioids-related food addictions, they are to be addressed at the psychophysiological level.

Issues with obesity and excess body fat

Reduced brain size
A research study conducted at Uppsala University in Sweden and published in the University's journal in early 2012 demonstrated that long-term obesity results in cognitive deficits because the brain regions that control appetite are altered in obese individuals. The study's findings have been published in the International Journal of Obesity.
http://www.uu.se/en/news/news-document/?id=1591&typ=pm&area=2&lang=en

Shorter life span
Morbidity and mortality has been studied in many cases where obesity and excess weight were problematic. Studies have shown that the death rate in overweight and obese people had doubled in numbers between 1993 and 2008.

Cognitive decline
European clinical studies continue to show and document poorer mental outcomes in obese people compared to non-obese ones.

Reduced quality of life
When it comes to physical and mental factors, they play an important role in everyone's quality of life. In overweight and obese people, there can be detectable signs of decreased function. When issues are compounded by depression, such people's quality of life can be affected in adverse ways.
http://psychcentral.com/news/2010/08/04/obesity-undermines-quality-of-life/16393.html

Higher rate of degenerative diseases
Overweight and obese people are at a much higher risk of developing the following health issues: hypertension, cancer, diabetes, rheumatoid arthritis, osteoarthritis, Parkinson's Disease, and prostatitis, among many more illnesses.

Psychosocial problems
Due to social stigmas and judgment experienced in relation to the weight and obesity impediments, affected people are likely to exhibit depression, addictions, overt and covert aggression, isolationism etc. They may feel a need for social withdrawal, due to: inability to fit into standard seats in public settings, (e. g. on airplanes), sleeplessness, excessive and loud snoring that may affect their relationships, erectile dysfunction, low libido, loss of physical appeal, erratic eating patterns, inability to participate in sports, skin problems, and in some cases, body odor, incontinence, etc.

Obesity and poverty

Usually, poor people cannot afford quality nutritious food. Given that some of the most obese people are also some of the poorest, there seems to be an obvious connection between low quality, deficient foods and the excess production of body fat. When the food supply of a malnourished individual is very toxic, their toxicity causes the body to experience a disturbance in the trigger system. This is the system that signals to the person when it is time to feel full at feeding time. When the signals are disrupted, overfeeding occurs due to insatiable frequent hunger that eventually causes stomach and abdominal distention in addition to excess body fat.

OBESITY RATE BY INCOME LEVELS

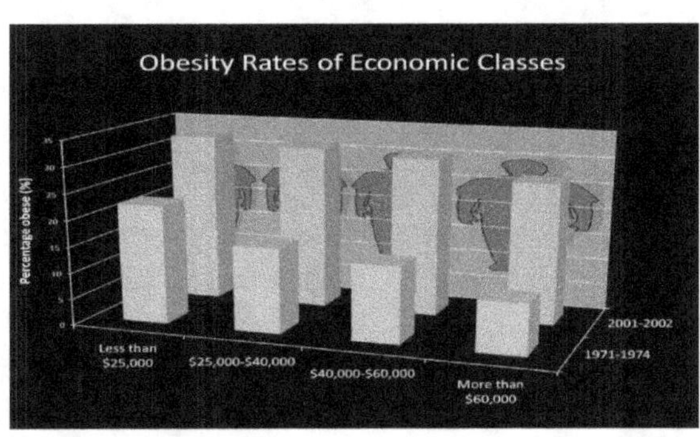

Source: commons.wikimedia.org

Importance of resolving issues by addressing their causes

Weight management is not about popping diet pills, wearing girdles, using a walking cane, and rolling in a wheelchair while perpetuating bad habits such as sipping diet soda. Proper weight control is all about investigating causes in order to find solutions to the effects. All causes are already uncovered; all effects are already understood. What to do next is making the connection between causes and effects, and applying the proper methodologies for damage control.

Useful resources:
1. CBS News :: Diane Sawyer interview with Dr. Marie Savard on soda consumption:
http://www.youtube.com/watch?v=P5tpCpqABhM
2. Reader's Digest :: Diet sodas: http://www.rd.com/health/diet-weight-loss/is-diet-soda-making-you-fat/
3. Mark Hyman, MD ::Does Drinking Soda Make You Fat: http://www.youtube.com/watch?v=nzJ6ZbQN9mY
4. Dr. Mercola :: Psychosis due to brominated oils in some sodas:
http://articles.mercola.com/sites/articles/archive/2012/01/11/brominated-vegetable-oil-in-us-soda.aspx

For levity:

A beggar walked up to a chubby woman on the street and exclaimed,
"Lady, I haven't eaten in a week."

"Wow!" exclaimed the zaftig woman, "I wish I had your will power."

Source: danworona.50megs.com

Chapter 12

Solutions to Physiological Toxicity

"The body is your temple. Keep it pure and clean for the soul to reside in."
~ B.K.S. Iyengar, Yoga: The Path To Holistic Health

Detoxification of the physical body

The body is a temple for the people who treat it as such. For those who opt to treat it like a municipal dumpster, then it will eventually act as what their owner chooses it to be. Unless the body is pure or purified, and acting in congruency with the mind, the person who resides inside that body is not likely to create the proper conditions to manifest a harmonious life.

If you do not take care of your body, where will you live?

There was a time when most average people thought that living a healthy lifestyle meant: eat anything they want, whenever they want, however they want, wherever they want. They thought they could consume all the junk food that they could stomach, with all the artificial food stuff advertised on TV. They also thought it was inconsequential to ignore all fruits and vegetables, then take a daily synthetic vitamin pill, and eventually chew on toxic gum to mask the stench of putrefying food in the intestines. They thought it was fun to be a couch potato, do compulsive TV viewing, occasionally exercise for a show, and then expect radiant health... Unfortunately the prevalence of degenerative diseases in our society has come to prove this lifestyle to be of great detriment to those who followed it. It has also come to constitute a wake up call.

Considering that there are millions of toxic contaminants in our air, water, food, and everything else, it is important to clear them out of the system. It takes months – and in many cases, years – to properly detoxify the body from abuses or impurities of the past. An unhealthy lifestyle is detrimental to health because the human body malfunctions when abused.

Nowadays, there are many people who are aware of the connection between fitness and better health, plus they are more in tune with their own body. Others are learning how to do it through various methods. They have come to realize that radiant health can be a reachable goal, even when the body is under assault. This mostly has to do with changing their lifestyle. As seen in our chapter on detoxification from environmental pollution, detoxifying the physical body is one of the main conditions to shedding excess weight and possibly recovering from certain types of illnesses. One of the keys to wholeness is the systematic decontamination from the major and minor sources of pollution, whether the pollution is visible or invisible.

Because toxicity is rather an abstract concept for a lot of people -- since it is neither visible nor palpable -- it is sometimes hard to grasp. When detoxification is pursued at the cellular and energetic levels – with emphasis put on the root causes – then the chances of experiencing optimum wellness are maximized.

In her book on the Regenetics Method: *Conscious Healing*, Sol Luckman states:

> *"From a cymatic or vibratory standpoint, disharmony is disease. The critical concept to grasp here is that all manifestations of disease, whether diagnosed as "physiological" or "psychological," result from disruption (in the form of toxicity or trauma) of the primary electromagnetic harmonies and rhythms contained in the auric fields and corresponding chakras ... These bioenergy centers have an intimate relationship with DNA that gives them direct regulatory access to all cellular functions. Therefore, if we can find a way to reset our bioenergy blueprint through harmonic resonance, we can go directly to the root of disease processes."*
> Source: Conscious Healing: Book One on the Regenetics Method, Pages: 27
>
> http://blog.gaiam.com/quotes/topics/toxicity

Detoxification is a multi-level task that involves knowledge of cause and effect, taking into consideration different levels of toxicity and knowing where the toxins reside. Detoxification also involves proactively addressing all underlying causes and eventually making lifestyle changes in order to yield desirable results.

The following is a summary of the detoxification steps covered in the previous chapters.

Detoxification from air pollution

Our air is alarmingly polluted nowadays. The number of airborne contaminants that are grounds for diseases is said to be on the rise. The number of such contaminants is measurable. People who think they are only paying for food and water are mistaken: we are also paying a high price for air, due to all the inconveniences caused by allergies and ailments caused by airborne pollution. In order to access presumably cleaner air, we require sophisticated air purifiers and yet, there is no guarantee that we are getting the benefits we are sold on.

Action steps for purifying the body from air toxicity:

1. Use a quality air purifier. Non-purified indoor air can be as polluted and at times more polluted than outdoors air.

2. Place purifying plants in various places in your space. Bamboo and other plants as referred to in the chapter on environmental detoxification. Indoor air purifying plants attract dust particles and may neutralize harmful contaminants.

3. Do thorough cleaning of your space with non-toxic ('green'), eco-friendly products.

4. Ventilate.

5. Cleanse the nasal passages with a simple saline solution made of distilled water and 3% salt. For those who wonder about *neti* pots, it is important to know how to use them properly and follow safety precautions relating to water sterilization and disinfection.

Detoxification from water pollution

Our water supply is in a serious state of contamination globally. Some rivers and bodies of water are becoming gradually extinct, due to excessive pollution caused by phosphates and other inorganic chemicals from cleaning products. There is a huge number of chemicals in our water supply; unfortunately, the world is currently not doing much to control the situation.

Action steps for purifying the body from water toxicity:

1. Purchase a quality water purification system or water filter. The cost of a good water filter is about the same as (and perhaps less than) a one to two-month supply of plastic bottled water.

2. Secure replacement filters for the water filter, just in case the filter stays inactive for a while, such as one month or so.

3. Avoid phthalates-contaminated bottled water.

Know certain facts about bottled water hazards:
1. Most bottled water is simply tap water mechanically put into a plastic bottle. The bottle itself has the potential for having hormone-disruptive toxins and cancer-causing chemicals leaching into the water and compounding the water's toxicity.

2. By the time you purchase bottled water, due to the plastic that contains it, such water is likely to have been contaminated by Bisphenol-A and phthalates that are known to cause degenerative illnesses, endocrine dysfunctions, and genetic mutations.

3. Bottled water is 10,000 to 100,000 times more expensive than tap.

4. While you are paying top dollars for additional contaminants from the plastic, your bottled water is no better than the tap that is already overly contaminated.

5. Replacing plastic bottles with glass is a safer way of storing drinking water.

Detoxification from food pollution

As seen earlier, most food pollution usually comes from:

- Airborne contaminants, unsanitary handling, pesticides, herbicides, fungicides, etc.
- Heavy metals.
- Plastic and chemical products that give off phthalates, Bisphenol-A, nano-technological particles, etc. (check chapter on environmental detoxification)
- Artificial additives, colorings, preservatives, etc.

It is not unusual to find toxic preservatives such as propylene glycol (antifreeze) in the food supply. It is present in ice cream, coconut flakes products, artificial vanilla, some commercial salad dressing products, and synthetic liquid vitamins, to name a few.

In 1991, while in college, a student once commented in a human nutrition class that some pasta noodles contained artificial food dyes. The professor, a registered dietitian, immediately snapped: *"That's not true!"* and the sneer on her face proved that she was asserting herself as a learned scholar, but not as a lifelong learner. Since then, the student began securing pieces of evidence: noodle packaging clearly showing on the label: FD&C Yellow # 5. At the time of this disagreement, prestigious universities had not yet done much research on the subject, therefore did not have such data in their textbooks. Artificial food dyes are proven carcinogens that have been found in noodles, pasta, and also macaroni and cheese products. Where superficial knowledge is bliss, it is easier to discredit than to do fact-finding. Check for research: http://en.wikipedia.org/wiki/Tartrazine

> *"In times of change, learners inherit the earth, while the learned find themselves beautifully equipped to deal with a world that no longer exists".*
>
> ~ Eric Hoffer

Action steps for purifying the body from food toxicity:

1. Properly hydrate the body by reasonably increasing your intake of pure water. The quality of the water is as important as the amount. There is no substitute for pure water.

2. Do a full body detoxification process with an integrative physician or nutritionist.

3.   Know what kind of produce is most heavily treated with pesticides and what type is treated the least. For the most recent list from the Environmental Working Group (EWG): http://www.ewg.org/foodnews/

4.   For personal knowledge and inspiration, there are manuals on detoxification such as:
     i.   ***Guide to Better Bowel Care: A Complete Program for Tissue Cleansing and Bowel Management*** by Dr. Bernard Jensen, a prolific writer and Chiropractor who lived until the ripe age of 93.
     ii. ***Detoxification: A Natural Approach***, by Gary Null. The book is a complete guide to cleansing the body and covers information ranging from juicing to colonics.

5.   Learn how to effectively juice fruits and also vegetables for proper detoxification.

"Some people have a foolish way of not minding, or pretending not to mind, what they eat. For my part, I mind my belly very studiously, and very carefully; for I look upon it, that he who does not mind his belly will hardly mind anything else."

~ Samuel Johnson

Detoxification from parasites

In case of parasitism, affected people must detoxify their level of hygiene to the maximum, both externally and internally. Professional help may be required.

Internally, a full body detox is necessary if one is serious about getting parasites under control, especially in case there is extra weight that may have been hard to manage.

Externally, in case of ringworm and fungi, an individual must fully detoxify and upgrade their personal lifestyle while finding appropriate solutions for eradication purposes.

Action steps for purifying the body from parasites toxicity:

1.   Wash one's hands often and meticulously.

2.   Wash bedding and towels regularly, at least weekly.

3.   Get the pets' bedding regularly sanitized.

4.   Do an internal cleanse for parasites control.

5.   Curb the ingestion of raw/undercooked meats and fish, unwashed fruits, sugar, unfiltered water, etc.

<u>Useful resources:</u>
Wholeness Connection: http://wholenessconnection.org (561) 767-1177 or (201) 242-0660
Video :: Parasites and the Brain: http://www.youtube.com/watch?v=R9hwmKQGPG0
An investigation of Toxoplasma Gondii and Schizophrenia

Detoxification from noise pollution

Our metropolises and megapolises are dreaded for their high levels of noise, from motorized traffic noise, electronic noise to noise from people and machinery. Inharmonious noise is a blatant form of pollution. It causes fatigue, psychological distress, and a whole host of emotional issues. Everything has a frequency, and so does noise. The likeliness of developing diseases in a noise-polluted environment is high because noise pollution adversely affects the immune system.

Action steps for shielding the body from noise toxicity:

1. Turn TV sets and radios off if there is no national or weather emergency.

2. Turn down ringers and alarm noises.

3. Use specific sound frequencies measured in hertz (Hz) that can also be utilized to counteract noise pollution.

4. Sound-proof one's personal space.

Detoxification from Electromagnetic Frequency (EMF) pollution and radiation

Action steps for shielding the body from EMFs and radiation:

1. Unplug TV sets, radio transmitters, and computers when not in use.

2. Keep electric and electronic devices away from the body as much as possible.

3. Use a Gauss meter to detect the areas of utmost concentration for the radiation.

4. Buy a radiation protection device. Electromagnetic frequency shields are known to offer required protection from EMF toxicity.

5. In serious cases of EMF toxicity, it can be of great help to use aluminum foil to line surfaces such as walls, ceilings, headboard, furniture, or anything that may be in direct contact with the source of radiation.

6. Avoid putting cellular phones in direct contact with the ear. Use earphones and an anti-radiation device. Aluminum foil also helps shield the body from the EMF emissions coming from cellular phones.

Detoxification from alcohol and drugs toxicity

In many people, when addiction has already been an issue for years, the longer the usage of addictive substances, the higher the risk of brain damage for the addicted person.

Action steps for purifying the body from alcohol and drugs toxicity:

1. Do a full body detox process with a holistic / integrative physician or nutritionist.

2. Ask the physician or nutritionist about homeopathic formulas used to stabilize the emotional states negatively influencing the physical body.

3. Ask the physician or nutritionist about a food supplementation program. Often, toxic and addicted people suffer from nutrient deficiencies that aggravate their addictions.

4. Enroll in a 12-step program for addictions.

Detoxification from dry cleaning residues

Mike Adams, the Health Ranger from NaturalNews.com has reported: *"In 1996, the National Institute for Occupational Safety and Health conducted a study to determine the hazards of PERC to dry cleaning workers. They determined that long-term exposure to PERC increased risk of cancers and other diseases. But what about consumers who simply want their clothing dry cleaned? Environment, Health and Safety Online reports that repeated exposure to high levels of PERC (and possibly even lower levels) can cause adverse effects. Many people note when they take their dry cleaning out of the bag, they smell a sweet, sharp scent: that's PERC, and that smell means they have been exposed."*

Learn more: http://www.naturalnews.com/030790_dry_cleaning_health.html#ixzz2IwAwJa00

Action steps for purifying the body from dry cleaning toxicity:

1. Do a full body detox process with an integrative physician, nutritionist, or natural hygienist.

2. Use a green dry cleaning facility. Even if green, air out the dry cleaned garments for at least 24 hours before wearing them.

3. Ensure that the service from the dry cleaning facility is truly green / eco-friendly.

Detoxification from all other contaminants

As covered earlier, regarding unseen, unproven, and unrecognized contaminants, it is essential to do a full body detoxification regardless of the nature of the pollutants.

Ancient natural therapies for additional detoxification

Skin brushing: A process that helps to detoxify the skin, control cellulite, and relieve stress due to its nurturing effect on the adrenals. It is performed with a dry brush made of soft natural bristles, on dry skin, for approximately five minutes.

Herbal baths therapy: Used in Indigenous and European medicines, they can pull toxins out of the body through the pores and promote healing through the absorption of healing essential oils from the herbs. Dead Sea salts or magnesium sulfate (Epsom Salt) may be added to the bath to help potentiate its effects and re-mineralize the system.

Bentonite clay baths: They are capable of detoxifying the body from heavy metals such as mercury. They were often used for skin care in ancient Rome and Greece.

Sulfur baths: They have been used for thousands of years in different cultures to detoxify and control health ailments from skin issues and chronic pain to urinary tract infections.
http://www.umm.edu/altmed/articles/sulfur-000328.htm
Sulfur springs can be of great benefit to some ailing people. Throughout the world, spas offer such commodities; some are naturally-occurring, and others are man-made.

Sauna: While some people may think that accessing a sauna is a European indulgence or an expensive proposition, exposure to a sauna can help detoxify toxic people successfully and quickly. Most quality spas have a sauna; many people also have their own sauna at home. Saunas are sold either as permanent fixtures or portable equipment.

Massage therapy: It is a popular form of energy medicine. There are different types of massage modalities, some of which are:
. Shiatsu (meridian-based massage) also known as Acupressure.
. Swedish.
. Deep tissue.
. Lymph drainage
. Reflexology (face, hands, and feet).
. Tui Na (Chinese massage).

Massage therapy can be quite detoxifying when properly performed.

Aromatherapy: It uses pure essential oils distilled from plants to promote specific effects, from anxiety relief and mental clarity, to pain relief and appetite control.

Exercises: In moderation, they protect from illness and prolong lives if already ill.

Upgrading one's nutrition for maximum detoxification

The food supply is loaded with hidden processed sugar, mostly high fructose corn syrup, which is one of the main causes of obesity, excess body weight, and diabetes. It is important to eat more like a hunter-gatherer and proceed to the systematic phasing out of processed foods.

DAILY ESSENTIALS FOR PROPER NUTRITION		
Food	**Daily Quantity**	**Benefits**
Water	6 to 8 or more glasses a day, depending on body size and bladder capacity. A recommended measure is 50 oz per pound of body weight.	Flushes out toxins and reduces acid in the body. Helps maintain the skin and keep bowels functional.
Fruits	2 or more – Reduce if a diabetic.	Beneficial fiber, vitamins, minerals, enzymes, good carbs for energy.
Vegetables	3 to 5 or more	Beneficial fiber, phytochemicals, minerals, enzymes, unprocessed carbs.
Starch carbohydrates	1 serving per meal	Help maintain energy levels.
Protein	1 serving per meal	Helps maintain muscle mass
Fats	1 to 3 tablespoons	Provide essential fatty acids necessary to keep the colon and joints lubricated, the skin healthy and hair soft and shiny.
Phytochemicals	1 to 3 servings of herbal teas such as: green tea, chlorophyll, Spirulina, etc.	Detoxify at the cellular level.

A sensible wellness formula for wholeness of body and mind

Detoxification (Tissue Cleansing and Hydration) + Replenishment = Wellness
Wellness + Environmental + Psychological + Spiritual balance   = Wholeness

Hydration through the proper ingestion of pure water is a very important step in obtaining and maintaining wellness of body and mind.

For levity:

"The way he treated his body, you would think he was renting it."

~ Robert Brault

Part III

PSYCHOLOGICAL TOXICITY

<h1 style="text-align:center">Chapter 13</h1>

<h1 style="text-align:center">Causes and Effects of Psychological Toxicity</h1>

"It's easy to believe that toxins are assaulting us on all fronts, but the worst toxins are often within. Worry is a toxin, envy is a toxin, self-loathing and fear and free-floating anxiety are all poisonous to our health"

~ Anna Johnson

Psychological Toxicity

For millennia, Chinese medicine has recognized the connection between human emotions and their effects on the physical body. Western medicine has only recently come to acknowledge such a connection. This acknowledgment has then opened the way for the fields of Neurobiology (also Neuroscience) and Psychoneuro-immunology, among many others. In Chinese medicine, there are seven fundamental emotions that play a major role in the function of the physical body: anger, grief, over-excitement, sadness, fear, worry, and terror.   Systematic deterioration of bodily organs occurs when the emotions are out of balance, exacerbated, or out of control.

Psychological toxicity is one of the three main factors responsible for mental disorders. As far as the three factors are concerned, they have been established as:

1. Biological.
2. Psychological.
3. Environmental.

Within the biological factors, there are sub-factors that are listed as:

1. DNA damage due to trauma (from prenatal to adult trauma, and other factors).
2. Brain defects.
3. Injuries to the brain or neurological system.
4. Bacterial infections.
5. Nutrition deficiencies / Addictions / Chemical imbalances.

There is a noted correlation between negative emotions and organs toxicity:

Anger

Also expressed as rage, frustration, and resentment, it adversely and mainly affects the liver on an energetic level. Over the long run, it has negative repercussions on the heart.

Grief

Also expressed as despair, it causes afflictions of the lungs and eventually the heart. In Chinese medicine, heart function co-depends on lung function.

Terror

Also expressed as shock and fright, it brings illness to the gallbladder, kidneys, and eventually the heart.

Over-Excitement

Also an expression of manic behavior, it adversely affects the heart. The one who is overly excited is likely to be overly depressed in the next hour or so (bi-polar traits).

Sadness

Also expressed as despondency, sadness damages the lungs and heart.

Fear

Also an expression of dis-empowerment, fear causes issues that perturb the kidneys.

Worry

Also expressed as excessive thinking, worry negatively influences the spleen and heart.

Negative emotions and low vibrational frequencies

Humans express their emotions through words and body language. People who do not have enough maturity to control their emotions often get stuck in a wavelength of negativity that makes them and their environment toxic.

In his book entitled ***Power vs. Force***, David R. Hawkins, MD, Ph.D., a healing psychiatrist, demonstrates the correlation between human behavior and its corresponding levels of consciousness. Dr. Hawkins' Scale of Consciousness, calibrates emotions on a scale of 1 to 1,000. The scale is a useful tool that can help to determine where individuals or groups fit with respect to their levels of consciousness. The book has pertinent data that assists one in learning how to instantly determine truth from falsehood. On the scale, shame ranges at 20, fear and grief at 75, while courage ranges at 200. Acceptance ranges at 350 and joy at 540. The highest scores on the scale are peace at 600 and enlightenment at 700-1,000.

When people enjoy the benefit of functioning at a higher level of consciousness, it is easier to interact with them because of the focus on respect and harmony. It is the lower forms of consciousness that are unfortunately stuck into a negative spiral that do not seem to easily or willingly respond to the call for higher evolution.

A simple observation of city dwellers as opposed to inhabitants of rural areas can help with the understanding of the detriment of urban toxicity. The more dense the population, the more complex, inhumane, harsh, unhealthy – therefore toxic – the lifestyle. Such lifestyle usually has serious adverse implications on the mind and body, and as a result a lot of people have become more robot-like and virtually de-humanized, de-sensitized, and dangerous.

> *"The industrial revolution has tended to produce everywhere great urban masses that seem to be increasingly careless of ethical standards."*
>
> ~ Irving Babbit

The mind leads the body. Its conscious expression is manifested through thought. The mind of many humans is on a default setting. This default setting causes people to end up creating their reality as if by default, rather than by choice. This is a major cause for human sufferings. In our society, there is an obsessive focus on over-competitiveness, control, abuse of power, and deception. For a lot of people, this is considered to be normal human behavior. This mentality is toxic and stems from a contrived sense of lack. People share thought waves on many levels and replicate behavior unconsciously. That is why new trends are adopted so fast, whether they are good or bad. An honest look at the way commercial products are manufactured, advertised, and marketed can bring awareness on how toxic commercial mentality affects the populace.

The mental body

The mental body is connected to the intellect and the conscious mind. It is undeniable that in the case of psychosomatic illnesses, the mind arranges circumstances to create a very real impression of disease in the body. Many states of dis-ease start at the mental level and eventually take a stronghold on the physical body. This situation indicates that no amount of physical cure can effectively work for such conditions unless the issue is properly addressed at the mental level.

Unaddressed trauma can cause psychological toxicity to become exacerbated. When you are the one affected by psychological toxicity, if you are aware of it and capable of taking action to remedy the situation, it has to be done consistently, and ideally with the guidance of a qualified therapist, a mental health practitioner, or an experienced minister.

If you are dealing with others who are afflicted by psychological toxicity, it is a very difficult path to walk. The closer you are to the person, the more difficult it is to handle the situation. A lot of afflicted people are in denial about their condition. Their denial may also be expressed through fierce or stubborn resistance. For this reason, no amount of reasoning or coaxing can get such person to admit that they do have a problem and require professional help. If you happen to be the primary caretaker or companion of a toxic person, their toxicity may significantly affect you and decrease your quality of life. Chinese herbal medicine and homeopathy have various remedies for detoxification. They help with the clearing of blocked energetic pathways in a person.

The emotional body

The emotional body is connected to the subconscious mind. Emotions come into manifestation through speech. They are not easy to hide even though they can be manipulated with conscious effort and skills. They are a reliable gauge of what feelings we are processing. When our speech is inharmonious and hostile, it is a clear sign that we are processing toxic emotions.

Some people try to conceal their anger by faking harmonious behavior but usually end up in a passive-aggressive mode. Those who were repressed children who had experienced an overly strict or harsh upbringing know that they could avoid being punished if they appeared to be on their best behavior when they were angry. They have, over the years, become accustomed to passive- aggression instead of open hostility. In many cases, hiding true emotions helps in face-saving or survival situations. Regardless of how convenient it may seem to conceal one's true emotions, this can be a dysfunctional coping style that often ends up causing various psychosomatic illnesses. When our coping mechanisms are inadequate, we develop a sense of frustration and helplessness that eventually compounds the existing emotional disorders.

Causes of psychological damage

Different types of psychological damage can occur in some people due to certain factors, some of which can be identified as:

- Childhood trauma, child abuse, neglect, brutality, abandonment, etc.
- Abuse (physical, sexual, psychological, etc.)
- Chemical drugs.
- Exposure to combat, domestic violence, shock.
- Malnutrition, nutritional deficiencies, chemical imbalances, addictions.
- Innate failure programs.
- Implants.
- Psychological control devices.

Effects of psychological damage

When people experience psychological damage, it often expresses itself in the form of imbalances. A few of them are known as:

1. Post Traumatic Stress Disorder (PTSD): a severe form of anxiety disorder that some individuals develop after exposure to a life threatening, traumatic event. PTSD sufferers function within chaos and sometimes do not want any structured order in their life. Chaos is often the default setting. PTSD affected people often resort to the escapism of addiction.

2. Attention Deficit Disorder / Attention Deficit Hyperactivity Disorder (ADD/ADHD): they are trauma-based disorders causing people to be unable to focus their attention on simple tasks that non-affected individuals usually accomplish automatically.

3. Cognitive dissonance: holding two conflicting sets of beliefs, a situation that eventually causes confusion and denial.

4. Personality disorders: issues known as narcissism, compulsive behavior, borderline personality disorder, antisocial behavior, and more. They involve emotional instability.

During the formative stages of life, any type of abuse can end up being conducive to psychological trauma. It comprises, ill-care, neglect, physical, sexual, and psychological abuse, etc. People who have had an abusive childhood are likely to repeat the patterns of abuse later in their own life and with their offspring. Pre- adulthood abuse usually leads to:

Self-Abuse
People who are energetically imbalanced abuse of themselves quite unconsciously: bad diet, smoking, drinking, physical and psychological self-abuse. They often have recourse to alcohol, drugs, or medications to numb the psychological pain they find unbearable.

Abuse of others
It is a parent who has been abused by their own parent(s) that usually ends up abusing their children, and/or their mate and everybody else. There are people who abuse children because they feel dirty and have been abused by other people. It is the nature of people that have been shamed to dump their shame somewhere. They use children because children have much less emotional baggage than adults. Some devious people find it easier to control a child through bribes and lies than they can control an adult.

Abandonment issues
Either real or perceived, abandonment can carry severe and permanent consequences in a child; this usually represents a condition that persists throughout the rest of people's adult life. If a child has experienced abandonment, later in their adult life, they are likely to have dysfunctional reactions toward anyone who is perceived as abandoning them. Abandonment issues can be so difficult to handle that some people may never recover.

Victimization
It involves the belief that one is trapped in a maladaptive paradigm. It leads to repeat patterns of the situations in which one has been, or felt victimized. It usually comes with low self-esteem, chronic depression, rage, inability to make choices, etc. A sense of victimization also leads to dis-empowerment, a state of mind characterized by a pronounced sense of despair and helplessness which can feel paralyzing for the mind. Victimization issues often cause people to turn their toxic emotions against themselves and against others who may not be the ones who have harmed them.

Mis-managed anger
It involves lashing out to express one's displeasure about certain challenges. It also leads to dis-empowerment. Basically, all humans have specific anger programs. Some of such programs have prenatal and precognitive causes. There is a major problem when anger turns chronic and when it is repressed. The act of repressing anger causes the state of anger to worsen due to the principle that repressed emotions usually reappear in other places and situations when one least expects that to happen. When the repressed emotions make their reappearance, they usually backfire and return with accumulated levels of energies that compound the original issue. This consequently makes the condition even more complex in its management and resolution, especially when the anger is turned against other people who may be used as scapegoats.

People who face issues of shame, guilt, fear, and inadequacies are usually plagued by feelings of anger and anxiety. In general, at some point in time, they experience psychosomatic illnesses and all types of imbalances such as sleep disturbances, eating disorders, sexual dysfunction, lack of self- control, etc. They act impatiently with the people around them, push themselves illogically hard, and end up living an out of control life, with memory loss issues, uncontrolled rage, and chronic disasters. Eventually they end up with excess production of acid in their system and may develop health issues such as acid reflux, ulcers, kidney stones, liver disease, overweight conditions, obesity, to name a few.

For levity:

"The statistics on sanity are that one out of every four Americans is suffering from some form of mental illness. Think of your three best friends. If they seem ok to you, then you are the mentally ill one..."

~ Anon

Chapter 14

Solutions to Psychological Toxicity

*"In reality, a mind on overload is a sick mind, a toxic mind.
It must be alleviated before it can be repaired."*

~ Zarcharty Bercovitz

Being exposed to what most people call 'the real world' or 'real life' is usually a factor that can contribute to psychological toxicity. Between the ever-present bad news in the mainstream media and the energy of individuals vibrating at lower frequencies, it is quite easy to be psychologically contaminated. The tragedy is that many people equate chaos with 'the real world'.

We may choose to keep ourselves purified to a certain extent, however, being in frequent or close contact with more toxic beings can cause us to experience rebound energetic disturbances. To remedy the situation, it is in our best interest to detoxify ourselves mentally or emotionally on a regular basis in order to recover our own balance. The kind of toxicity transmitted from one person to another can be physical, emotional, psychological, mental, and more. The thoughts we process within ourselves play a major role in our lives. They influence the kind of people and circumstances we attract to ourselves. This kind of attraction is based on certain thought frequencies that eventually begin to resonate with us as vibrational matches because we may have consciously or unconsciously tuned in to them.

If you are unhappy in your body or home, are ill or depressed, detoxification is to begin at the level of the mind in order to be of benefit to the whole body. If you do not start repairing yourself at the level of the mind, any physical action you may take might end up being cosmetic and counterproductive in the long run.

Proper detoxification of the psychological body is a multi-dimensional process that includes:

Detoxification of the mental body.
Detoxification of the emotional body.
Detoxification of the soul body.

Left brain versus whole brain issues

Society trains us to use more of our left brain hemisphere than our right brain hemisphere. Our left brain is logical/rational, structured, memory and language-related. Our right brain is intuitive, non-verbal, feelings-oriented, and artistic. Using more of one side of the brain than the other presents the disadvantage of making us imbalanced. To reach wholeness and be in balance, it is important to utilize both hemispheres of the brain as equally as humanly possible.

Certain cultures are aware that society's emphasis on left-brain orientation may serve a specific purpose – that of a control program. Sometimes living within a system or a paradigm that demands blind and unquestioned obedience to authority figures entails accepting to play the manipulation program. Most people cooperate with the program in order to survive. When the right brain is fully activated, humans are more capable of utilizing their intuitive faculties and can afford enough insight to see through hidden agendas. It is through the pituitary and pineal glands that our inner vision and intuition are activated. Totalitarian systems often discourage right brain activity as an effort to prevent people from experiencing higher awareness. Usually, this discouragement takes place through fear and intimidation.

The Mind-Body Connection

Psychophysiology advocates treating the mind as well as the body. For instance, if someone has issues with their weight, nutrition alone may not fully help if the pent-up emotions causing emotional eating are not properly addressed. Inversely, physical conditions due to an accident or congenital defect may greatly affect someone's emotional state. To take it further, if we look beyond the accident, we discover that a person's emotional state may bring about the conditions that can cause accidents. All is inter-connected and must be addressed within appropriate context.

Candace Pert, Ph.D., a best-selling author, world-class neuroscientist, and research professor in the Department of Physiology and Biophysics at Georgetown University Medical Center in Washington, D.C. has stated:

> *"Most psychologists treat the mind as disembodied, a phenomenon with little or no connection to the physical body. Conversely, physicians treat the body with no regard to the mind or the emotions. But the body and mind are not separate, and we cannot treat one without the other."*

The following chapters cover information on how to detoxify the mental, emotional, and spiritual bodies each on different levels, using whole brain methodologies and energy therapies.

For levity:

> *"Just because you aren't paranoid doesn't mean they aren't out to get you! It's worse when you think they're out to get you!"*

> ~ Anon

Chapter 15

Detoxification of the Mental Body

"Our mind can either be our best friend or our worst enemy depending on what we feed it."
~ Anon

Akin to a sponge, the mind is highly permeable. It is capable of absorbing, processing, and retaining the essence of words, spoken or unspoken; it also resonates with frequencies whether they are detectable or not. Absorption and resonance can have their effect on the mind for extended periods of time and even forever. In computer language, GIGO is an acronym for 'Garbage In - Garbage Out'. The term applies to computers, as well as the mind and body.

The levels of frequencies that people's minds are exposed to, determine their attitudes and states of health or disease. The events people experience in their lives are the result of the thought frequencies they resonate with. Those who get most of their intellectual programming from indoctrination-based institutions and the media are likely to end up with pineal gland calcification. This causes a one-track mind situation and inhibits the ability to look at matters from different angles. Eventually, people end up regurgitating what they have been programmed with. This comes with the additional inconvenience of being extremely opinionated while exhibiting very little regard for objectivity. Additionally, people of this type tend to act as if they were the thought police, censuring and punishing anybody who thinks differently.

The mind rules the physical body. Its conscious expression is manifested by way of thought processes. The mental body is connected to the intellect and the conscious mind. It is through the conscious mind that we are aware of the physical world that we live in and the things that exist around us.

Our mental body is associated with our capacity to think, comprehend, and analyze data that is necessary in order for us to be fully functional beings. Whereas the emotional body starts its development in the first weeks of life, the mental body only starts developing around puberty.

112

Because body and mind are connected, our different states of mind do influence the physical body. From a psychosomatic point of view, since the mind greatly influences the body, many states of dis-ease start at the mental level, before they take a stronghold on the physical body. This situation entails that in most cases, no amount of cure can effectively work to heal the physical body from the condition unless the issue is properly addressed at the mental level.

~Thomas Wolfe

Issues with toxic mental overload

A large number of mental conditions stem from mental overload from various stressors. Humans think between 20,000 and 70,000 thoughts daily. Some people may be affected by stressors and not quite be aware of them. This is particularly true if they are used to a high stress environment where multiple stress factors come into play, or if they are not very aware or attentive to their own body. Just about everyone seems to be on some sort of mental overload nowadays. The majority of the people who have to work for a living are usually stressed out. People who, not only work to make a living, but also are pursuing an education and / or are raising a family are on maximum overload. Because of the issue of overload that seems to be a prevailing factor in many people's lives nowadays, it is obvious that for the sake of maintaining or recovering one's sanity, the first priority should be to reduce toxic overload. Some recovering toxicity addicts are able to accomplish a release of mental overload by curbing the intake of all external data that is neither essential to their livelihood nor relevant to their survival.

One of the major problems with mental overload is that when a person keeps bottling up stress and negative emotions, over time, they become a toxic time bomb. The ready-to-detonate bomb may explode in the most negative of ways any time, harming other people and self-destructing in the process. When the issue is not properly or professionally addressed, it can lead to serious problems such as psychosocial crises. For instance, on many occasions, some people have 'gone postal', meaning they have taken their anger out on postal employees and patrons. They got inside the post office and went on a killing rampage. In all cases of toxic emotional overload or un-managed personal distress, the person experiencing the problem must have it properly addressed through effective methods of rehabilitation. Such methods are numerous, available everywhere at any time, and they work. It is the lack of management of personal toxicity that usually causes people to be a hazard to themselves and others. One of the main reasons for mental overload is excessive exposure to negative mental programming.

Issues with toxic mental programming

The mind of many humans is, on many levels, on a default setting. Most people end up creating their reality by default rather than by choice; this situation is one of the most major causes of human sufferings. The mind of people can be controlled through fear, drama, and repetition.

The repetition works, and this is why media advertising, propaganda, and mainstream indoctrination have such an effective impact on their audience. Repetitions play an important role in anchoring verbal command. For example, when people are often exposed to commercials that claim certain benefits to a product, even if the claims are inauthentic, people are likely to buy and consume the product repeatedly. The media in many ways represents an authority figure to people. At times, some people may find out that a product is bad for them, but they will consume it anyway because, once again, the media promotes it. There is an overwhelming number of packaged food and beverages, fast food products, toxic cleaning products, and personal care products advertised in the media. There is, however, very little industry accountability regarding the increasingly number of toxic, ill, and out of shape people.

Toxic effects of excessive television viewing

When people watch television programs, they may find it to be an entertaining, informative, or educational experience. There are channels such as the History Channel, that present informative and educational materials in an entertaining way. Television programs can offer a way to relax however, in general, a program may also entail what it is meant to be: a program that is intended to work on programming the viewer's mind. When it comes to the news, it can be entertaining for some people however, most of the news involve a detailed, graphic display of every accident, murder, criminal activity, mishaps, dire predictions, anything from adverse weather conditions to economic downturn, etc. If you listen to the news occasionally so as to be informed about a major event, there is some benefit to that. However, to make news programming a daily staple and allowing the self to absorb the programming either at meal times or sleep time is toxic. Sleeping for many hours with toxic programming on contributes to detrimental health effects over time. In what sense is the repeated mental imagery of every murder, every accident, every crime, every shooting, helping one live a wholesome life?

The mind processes information sent to it through sound, images, ultra-sonic frequencies, and other means. Data we are exposed to right before we fall asleep is what our mind processes throughout our sleep time. Many people complain of insomnia, nightmares, and night terrors. Most of them take medications for sleep disorders . Not all people make the connection between the self-imposed pre-sleep programming and their sleeplessness issues. As seen above, the mind processes information during sleep and when one sleeps with the horror movie on, what does the mind process? Usually people do not remember the specifics of the program when they were exposed to it, but they know that they did not sleep well. Those who leave their TV on while they sleep are also processing on a subliminal level whatever data is encoded in the program. There are subliminal messages in a lot of programs. Most of them are geared toward implanting in the viewer's mind suggestions that they need to buy products. A lot of the time, the show itself is not something that knowledgeable viewers would consider to be wholesome.

TV programming often features covert subliminal messages suggesting that the viewer needs or wants to consume some advertised products, many of which usually include processed foods. Over time, the viewer starts to believe that their life will improve through speed and convenience if they consume the goods and keep up with the Joneses.

The problem with the suggestions to consume toxic products is that what one gains in speed and convenience, one loses in terms of quality of health. A lot of the cleverly advertised products shown in the media are presented in ways that lull the public into thinking that they are indispensable. This is done under the guise of promising to improve people's lives but in general, the products are loaded with toxic chemicals. Additionally, there are subliminal suggestions that convince the viewer to obey hidden commands. Research studies have found a correlation between TV viewers' habit of falling asleep with the TV on and their urges to consume the processed foods that have been advertised. The situation is dire for shopaholics who fall asleep with their TV on.

Because TV viewing is not interactive, it has been found to thwart its frequent viewers' ability to get their brain faculties properly stimulated. Non-interactive viewing rather encourages mental dullness due to extreme and prolonged relaxation that is unproductive. This dullness of the mind is designed to promote extreme passivity and docility. This, in addition to the covert mental manipulations embedded in the advertisements, promotes the eventual acceptance of everything that is presented through the medium as "truth". People accept this perceived "truth" although it is deceptive, unethical, or misinformative.

Toxicity serves an understated purpose of preventing us from accessing our right brain faculties. When such faculties are fully functional, we are more capable of living free from excessive consumerism. We are also less subjected to the assaults of a *weaponized* and toxic lifestyle. Any paradigm that discourages the use of right brain and whole brain functions has a long-term agenda that is not necessarily in our best interest. Additionally, excessive TV viewing has been found to cause excess stress to the pineal gland and put the mind on overload.

There is a very fine demarcation line between the mental and the emotional aspects of the body. Even though the two may be so closely interlinked that their characteristics overlap, the differences between them do exist so that bodily functions may occur in a subtle manner.

Humans do transmit energetic frequencies to each other mentally. Here are some examples of how the transmission usually happens:
1. The music track we heard someone sing may stay on repeat mode in our memory for hours or longer.
2. The tears of sadness we see someone shed in front of us may instantaneously cause us to start shedding tears also.
3. The anger someone expresses toward us may cause us to echo it back to the person and then project it onto others too.
4. The exciting words of someone telling us about a new promising project may fill us with joyful anticipation and eagerness for a while.

Because we are so connected to each other on a vibratory level, it is important to keep one's frequency high on the vibratory scale. That can allow us to muster the strength it takes to counteract any low vibrations we are very likely to encounter. This can help preserve our sanity.

If you are unhappy in your body or home, if you are ill or depressed, it might be a sign that perhaps it is time that you start a detoxification process. Begin with detoxifying the mind in order to get the purification to benefit to the whole body. It is necessary to begin repairing the self at the level of the mind; if any action that one takes is not in congruency with mental detoxification, it may just end up being a cosmetic and counterproductive effort, particularly in the long run.

Therapies that benefit the mental body

Mainstream therapists and energy therapists alike use different psychotherapeutic modalities to help resolve issues relating to psychological toxicity.

Psychotherapy

It is based on dialogue, behavior modification, self-discovery, and self-motivation. This therapy encourages constructive action for the purpose of recovering from trauma and dysfunction that may be impeding someone's life. It requires the intervention of a trained psychotherapist. There are different models of psychotherapeutic intervention. They are quite effective and many of them are complementary to each other. Some of them are:

Core Belief Process
It addresses negative emotions and limiting beliefs.

Rational Emotive Behavior Therapy (REBT)
Developed by Albert Ellis, Ph.D, REBT it is known to effectively assist in eradicating irrational behavior and fears to empower a person facing adversity.

Cognitive Behavior Therapy (CBT)
Similar to REBT, Cognitive Behavior Therapy uses mindfulness techniques in the management of toxic emotions associated with eating disorders, addictions, maladaptive patterns, anxiety, and depression.

Hypnotherapy
A popular modality that uses progressive relaxation to access subconscious states of mind to facilitate the programming or de-programming of the mind for specific purposes e.g. fear eradication or smoking cessation. Some therapists use related techniques such as regression therapy and parts therapy to clear specific maladaptive patterns.

Psychotherapeutic Energy Therapies

Emotional Freedom Technique (EFT)
An energy therapy modality that uses tapping on specific meridian points on the body in conjunction with other re-patterning modalities such as neuro-linguistic programming and re-framing for constructive change.

The Healing Codes
Alex Lloyd, Ph.D., N.D., a doctor of Naturopathic medicine and energy therapist is the creator of a self-healing system called The Healing Codes. When exposed to the Codes, people get a sense of self-empowerment that is conducive to their healing. The system also comes with a self-assessment technique that can be a true eye opener which motivates people to make the necessary changes in their life. In a recent presentation entitled *"What Have You Lost?"*, Dr. Lloyd explained:

"We've all lost something. What has it cost us?
A maladaptive sense of loss offers a very toxic environment for the development of a love relationship. Control, anger, impatience, mistrust, all contribute to stifling the relationship.

Every kind of relationship problem comes from a sense of loss. Whatever we have lost or what someone in our ancestry or relative has lost and has affected us. So many people are defined by the things they have lost and are stuck there. It's a closed door, off limit issue when you want to help them. They rationalize what they don't want to face. The memory of having something that you no longer have because it was of value to you.

Pornography is epidemic today, It is becoming more and more so in a lot of men and women. People who are addicted to pornography actually prefer it over normal actual relationships. They don't have the feeling of loss or rejection if someone in the porn is not attracted to them. It's on command, so they think it is within their control. If we don't deal with these issues of what we've lost, the destructive habits and addictions prevail. Narcissism also is what they use to imagine themselves being an imaginary successful being. The dark side of just imagining how amazing things are coming to them, it turns destructive. They are taking an ownership of an imaginary being. They feel in control. They think they are the person that all the girls are after. It has nothing to do with truth and love. When it doesn't happen in reality, they end up with a sense of loss and become stuck.

Some people can heal but they may not want to heal, and not be ready. There is a very famous entertainer who is stuck at the age of 6, which corresponds to when his father died. He's been offered to heal through therapy but he's always refused. His dysfunction has become his identity.

If you have one area of loss you will tend to respond to a program and do something pleasurable to be distracted which turns to an addiction over time. We should not be defined by the things we have lost or what we have. Those who had a high school reputation sometimes never recover from it. They still live as the fictitious football star or high school bully. They sometimes define themselves by their achievements. We should only be defined by our true identity: by love and by helping. Love more and deeper. Be more committed to the truth and to living in the present.

Mind clearing methods

In the age of toxic mental overload, we take in and process a whole load of data, some of which we do not need because it contributes neither to our livelihood nor our happiness. It is important to learn to unload and release toxic data that keeps being mentally processed long after intake and often results in stress-related disorders. Meditation and image streaming are known to help:

Meditation
It is an age-old practice that requires systematic relaxation of the body and mind to achieve stillness. It is the art of de-focusing on mundane thoughts to be receptive to inner insight. It has been scientifically proven to help individuals afflicted by high blood pressure, anxiety, and several other issues. It can help clear negative emotions.

Guided Imagery
It consists of relaxing the body and mind while following specific instructions from a live therapist or recording. By letting the mind free flow and let go of stress or mental burdens, useful imagery usually occurs.

Brain Wave Entrainment Technology

It is a technology that uses sounds, music, monaural and binaural beats to train the brain to produce more neurons and adopt specific patterns conducive to healthier states of mind. Neurons or neural pathways help increase emotional IQ.

Homeopathic Remedies

Homeopathic remedies are safe pharmaceutical-grade preparations that offer a whole range of different formulas for anything from colds and flu symptoms to emotional distress including PTSD. They are best used under the guidance of a trained homeopathic physician.

Mindfulness practice

So many of us are on mental overload that we are for the most part in mindlessness mode. This situation causes most of us not to care, not to be present for others and ourselves, and all that compounds any level of existing toxicity.

When we practice mindfulness, we make a conscious effort to be aware that first of all, we exist; second of all, we exist for a purpose; third of all, this purpose has to benefit others around us for our lives to be truly meaningful. When we are at that level, then we start paying attention to becoming aware of everything we do and say. We then make sure that what we do is benevolent for us and for the good of all that is around us, and that includes people, things, and our environment.

Yoga

Among various ancient techniques of self-actualization, yoga is one of the most widely practiced in the world. The reason for yoga's enormous popularity is because, as an effective but simple practice, it is based on the union of the mind, body, and emotions. It is this unification that translates into wholeness.

Brain foods

They assist in experiencing better focus and calmness of mind due to the input of quality nutrients they introduce into the body. When the body is given what it needs, it repairs itself at the cellular level. Some brain foods are readily available in supermarkets and health food stores. They are high in anti-oxidants, phytochemicals, vitamins, minerals, proteins, and adequate amounts of fat. Some of them are: Berries (Gogi berries, blueberries, strawberries, etc.), nuts and seeds, Greek yogurt, eggs, beans (kidney beans, soybeans, etc.), fish, hemp protein, Spirulina, and green tea. Soybeans, however, have estrogenic properties.

Full mind-body detox

The physical detoxification process is also helpful in ridding the mental body of toxins that may have affected it. Brain fog and confusion may be signs that toxins in the physical body are affecting mental functions. Toxic foodstuff and personal care products such as toxic shampoos and other hair care products have the ability to adversely affect the mental body.

Useful resources:

The Healing Codes: http://www.thehealingcodes.com/cmd.php?af=1515004

Brain Wave Entrainment Technology: http://www.mindpowermp3.com/idevaffiliate/idevaffiliate.php?id=1525

For levity:

"I believe in an open mind, but not so open that your brains fall out."

~ Arthur Hays Sulzberger

Chapter 16

Detoxification of the Emotional Body

"Your intellect may be confused, but your emotions will never lie to you."
~ Roger Ebert

Human emotions play a vital role in the body's functions. Words and body language are the vectors of emotions. Humans have a whole range of emotions encoded in them since the pre-natal stage. That is why babies can express pleasure, contentment, wonderment, frustration, separation anxiety, fear, and more.

The emotional body is associated with the ability to feel and communicate, either verbally, energetically, or through body language. It is in the first two years of life that the emotional body's development begins.

When someone is properly developed emotionally, they are endowed with the ability to be emotionally strong. This entails facing the difficulties of daily life with equanimity, an indicator of high emotional intelligence quotient, or emotional IQ. The characteristics of high emotional IQ are expressed through the ability to handle stress and conflict in a calm, in-charge, mature, and responsible way.

When emotionally immature people are challenged, their levels of agitation determine to what extent they perceive the challenge as a threat to them. The challenged individual sometimes reverts back to infancy or toddler mode as a coping strategy. Emotionally immature people are not wired to use their verbal skills or mental faculties to solve their issues when stressors pose a challenge to them. At times, you may see people dressed as professionals, carrying a briefcase to meetings, driving expensive cars, speaking in an articulate manner, but behaving like a rebellious two-year old. They often start lunging at others, out of control for the pettiest reasons. Even though they may look substantial, some of these individuals may be emotionally damaged, regardless of their professional status. Their behavior is often an indicator of when they may have experienced their first major trauma. The regression is usually expressed through fretting, screaming, pushing around, threatening, belittling, and eventually attacking. This type of person is rebellious by nature, is not self-governed but is not interested in self-control either.

For example, an individual may have the physical development of a 53-year old, the mental development of a 30 year-old, and the emotional maturity of a 2 year-old. Instead of managing their emotions, they let their emotions manage them when challenged. The most difficult types to deal with are narcissists, histrionics, borderline, antisocial, and bipolar people.

Seven toxic emotions and how to detoxify from them

<table>
<tr><td colspan="4" align="center">Seven Toxic Emotions</td></tr>
<tr><th>Emotions</th><th>Expressed as</th><th>Affects</th><th>Detoxify with</th></tr>
<tr><td>Anger</td><td>Rage, frustration, resentment</td><td>The liver</td><td>Full body detox with emphasis on liver cleanse, homeopathic remedies for anger, hypnotherapy, psychotherapy, anger management, lymphatic system cleanse.</td></tr>
<tr><td>Grief</td><td>Despair</td><td>The lungs, heart</td><td>Full body detox with emphasis on lungs cleanse, homeopathic remedies for grief and despair, hypnotherapy, psychotherapy, bereavement therapy, lymphatic system cleanse.</td></tr>
<tr><td>Terror</td><td>Shock and fright</td><td>The gallbladder, kidneys, heart</td><td>Full body detox with emphasis on gallbladder and kidney cleanse, homeopathic remedies for Post Traumatic Stress Disorder, hypnotherapy, psychotherapy, lymphatic system cleanse.</td></tr>
<tr><td>Over-excitement</td><td>An expression of manic traits</td><td>The heart</td><td>Full body detox with emphasis on lymph cleanse, homeopathic remedies for emotional imbalances, hypnotherapy, psychotherapy, anger management, lymphatic system cleanse, 528 Hz frequency.</td></tr>
<tr><td>Sadness</td><td>Despondency</td><td>The lungs and heart</td><td>Full body detox with emphasis on liver cleanse, homeopathic remedies for sadness, depression and despondency, hypnotherapy, psychotherapy, stress management, lymphatic system cleanse.</td></tr>
<tr><td>Fear</td><td>Dis-empowerment</td><td>The kidneys</td><td>Full body detox with emphasis on kidney cleanse, homeopathic remedies for fear, hypnotherapy, psychotherapy, anger, lymphatic system cleanse.</td></tr>
<tr><td>Worry</td><td>Excess pensiveness</td><td>The spleen and heart</td><td>Full body detox with emphasis on spleen detox , homeopathic remedies for worry, hypnotherapy, psychotherapy, lymphatic system cleanse.</td></tr>
</table>

Anger brings dis-empowerment. Humans have a huge amount of anger programs. When we repress anger, the matters we are angry about get compounded and worsen over time. The main problem with repressed emotions is that they usually reappear in other areas of life in unexpected ways that are as damaging and difficult to handle as when they are in their original state.

People who face issues of shame, guilt, fear, and inadequacies are usually plagued by feelings of anger and anxiety. In general, if these issues are not properly managed, soon the people are likely to experience psychosomatic illnesses and all types of imbalances such as sleep disorders, eating disorders, addictions, sexual dysfunction, and lack of self-control. Such people are likely to act with impatience with others around them, push themselves too hard, and end up living an out-of-control life. They often are in denial about their situation therefore, they have a tendency to shift blame often. Because it is hard for such individuals to face their own demise even when in denial, they usually end up with addiction issues, besides physical illness. Stress, when not properly handled, usually takes a toll on the physical and emotional bodies. In general, individuals develop coping mechanisms, some of which are more effective than others.

Some people have found the following approach to be useful in resolving emotional toxicity:

1. Self-confrontation regarding the origin, the root cause of the issue.
2. Self-analysis to bring awareness on the non-productivity of the toxic emotions.
3. Awareness of the rehearsal and entertainment of the said toxic emotions.
4. Self-acceptance and mindfulness exercises.
5. The practice of conscious detachment from the toxic behavior.

> *"Every good thought you think is*
> *contributing its share to the ultimate*
> *result of your life."*
>
> ~ Grenville Kleiser

Toxic people react differently from toxicity. Some people get a fix from toxins and some others exhibit symptoms that may cause them to experience discomfort. There are people who are so toxic that when exposed to a purified lifestyle, they exhibit symptoms that show evidence that their system is antagonistic to purity. Some other people repress or suppress their emotions and sooner than later, start functioning as toxic time bombs.

Resistance

One of the saddest things about toxic time bombs is their unwillingness to face their ordeal and their retreat into denial. They believe that by avoiding the issue and burying their head in the sand, they will go through life not feeling the pain of changing. What they are not aware of is the deep trail of pain they leave in the hearts of their family members, friends, colleagues, and acquaintances. Always, one can feel that the toxic person has great potential but such potential is either abused or left unexploited forever.

In spite of all of the therapeutic modalities that are available, many individuals do not want to be helped. They are programmed for failure. Even though a conscious part of them may be aware of the dysfunction or the damage, they falter. Although they may have some desire to improve, their subconscious programming may be too detrimentally potent to allow a shift. In spite of their best effort, these people will resist change and fight, postpone, or prevent their own healing.

> *"Resistance is thought transformed into feeling.*
> *Change the thought that creates the resistance, and there is no more resistance."*
>
> ~ Robert Conklin

Therapies that whole-brained therapists recommend for emotional detoxification

Hormonal balancing

In case one is experiencing frequent and uncontrollable mood swings that occur for no discernible reason, it is important to discuss the issue with a doctor of Integrative medicine or a doctor of Chinese medicine. There are natural hormone-balancing therapies that they may recommend. Mood swings can affect both middle-aged men and women, particularly when subjected to hormonal imbalances, blood sugar imbalances, adrenal exhaustion, nutritional deficiencies, etc.

Substance abuse treatment

In many cases, people get emotional or hostile due to withdrawal from drugs, alcohol, or smoking. In such cases, they are to seek help from rehabilitation facilities or from a hypnotherapist proficient at addictions cessation.

Inner Child healing

John Bradshaw, counselor, TV personality, and best selling author of several books and recordings is an expert on inner child healing. His material can be powerful in helping clear toxic emotions relating to past emotional trauma from childhood issues. It usually provides a cathartic experience with healing emotional issues concerning:

Abandonment
There are dire circumstances in life that cause people to resort to abandonment which hurts both the child and the parent. Recommended book/audio: "Homecoming – Reclaiming and Championing Your Inner Child".

Child abuse
It is an issue that affects countless people who remain silent because of fear and shame. Recommended books/audio: "Healing the Shame that Binds You" and also: " Incest and Sexual Addiction" (3-hr lecture on CD).

Addictions
People born of addicted parents usually end up becoming addicted and also pass the addictions to their own offspring. This cycle can be broken and the pattern discontinued once the dynamics are properly analyzed and comprehended. Recommended books/audio: "Healing the Shame that Binds You" and "A Theology of Addiction".

Eating disorders
It affects men and women alike and often has its roots in early childhood trauma of various kinds such as rejection, neglect, abandonment, gender issues, incest, etc. Recommended book/audio: "Eating Disorders" and "Healing the Shame that Binds You"

Emotional Freedom Technique (EFT)

EFT is an energy clearing method developed by Gary Craig. It involves a combination of affirmations in conjunction with finger-tapping on acupuncture-based trigger points corresponding to certain meridians in the human body. When using one's fingers to tap on the specifically designated points, one starts initiating a release process. The meridians one taps on relate to specific bodily organs which relate to certain emotions.

The following script can be used as a sample EFT tapping session. This particular script addresses the issue of emotional clearing.

EFT for Emotional Clearing

Karate Chop Point: "Even though I find it hard to control my emotions, I choose to accept myself nevertheless."

Inner corner of the eye: "Even though I sometimes experience self-destructive impulses that are stronger than my will, I choose to love and accept myself unconditionally anyway."

Outer corner of the eye: "Even though I feel like a victim of my circumstances, I choose to let go of this emotional burden and take my life back."

Under the Eye: "Even though I feel stuck at the age of   , I choose to let go of the past trauma and grow in wisdom and peace."

Under the Nose: "Even though I have been behaving in a way that no longer fits my age, I choose to remember that I can grow now because I am entitled to."

Chin: "Even though I am sometimes clueless about how self-destructive I am, I choose to change my behavior and clear myself from toxic emotions."

Collar Bone: "Even though this issue dis-empowered me, I choose to re-empower myself with love and respect."

Armpit: "Even though I have been feeling anxious out about this issue, I now make a conscious decision to release it."

Top of the Head: "Even though I sometimes feel truly overwhelmed about this issue, I choose to release the pain and take my life back nevertheless."

Heart: "And from now on, I choose to love and accept myself totally and unconditionally."

Parasitic organisms control

Candida cleanse

Candida albicans (yeast) overgrowth can contribute to emotional imbalances. They may adversely affect the internal organs, genitals, and brain function. Many people affected by candida find themselves on an emotional roller-coaster. Other indicators of candida overgrowth can be restlessness, irritability, brain fog, forgetfulness, nail fungus, vaginal discharge, and gastrointestinal issues, to name a few. The condition is often caused by over-consumption of sugar, yeast products such as bread, alcohol, smoked foods, and processed foods. In some cases, particularly when frequent alcohol and soft drinks consumption are involved, symptoms such as mood swings can be severe. Additionally one can incur a yeast overgrowth by using certain types of medications such as antibiotics that decrease friendly bacteria in the intestines. Negative attitudes can also contribute to candida proliferation. Yogurt consumption usually helps restore the colony of friendly bacteria.

Parasites cleanse

A lot of people who behave in mean and absurd ways are exhibiting symptoms of parasitic infestation. When affected by parasites, such as ascaris and oftentimes amoeba, someone's brain may be under assault. When it comes to mental dysfunction, parasites are not always tested for. Therefore, psychotropic drug therapy may not get to the core of the issue in case it relates to parasitism affecting the brain.

Hypnotherapy

It can assist in clearing negative blocks by accessing the subconscious mind. Certain techniques such as regression and parts therapy can be very useful for recovery from emotional disturbances.

Flowers and flower essences

They act at the subtle energy level. Their intrinsic beauty combined with their aroma and geometric shape are conducive to healing. When people are depressed or sick, flowers usually contribute to healing the emotions. That is why it is so comforting to have flowers around, in circumstances such as hospitalizations and funerals.

Reiki

A Japanese system of hands-on energetic healing that is used to balance mind and body. It is recognized as helping alleviate and even remedy blood pressure issues, emotional distress, anxiety, and stress. When combined with introspection Reiki is a method that can be effectively cathartic.

Therapeutic music

There is great therapeutic value in listening to healing sounds. In ancient Egypt and Babylon, sound frequencies combined with harmonic resonance and drumming were used to heal all kinds of health issues. Australian aboriginals still use *didgeridoo* sound frequencies for therapeutic purposes. Nowadays, Western medicine uses ultrasonic technology to address the issue of kidney stones.

Ho'Oponopono

It is a forgiveness-based Hawaiian Huna healing practice that consists of mindfully repeating four simple sets of words to obtain cathartic results when emotions are out of balance. The specific words are: *"I am sorry; please forgive me; thank you; I love you."*

Forgiveness

True forgiveness is one of the keys to compassion. It takes enormous practice in most cases. By accepting others, we forgive them and release ourselves, which initiates healing.

<u>**Useful resources:**</u>
1. Alcoholic home and maladaptive patterns: http://www.cmcsb.com/Living%20in %20an %20Alcoholic%20Home.html
2. Candida cleanse: http://www.candida30.net/candida30-program/?hop=pcg111
3. Parasites cleanse: http://www.livestrong.com/article/117883-herbs-cleanse-parasites/
4. Music therapy: http://www.mindpowermp3.com/idevaffiliate/idevaffiliate.php?id=1525

For levity:

"When people hurt you over and over, think of them like sand paper. They may scratch and hurt you a bit, but in the end, you end up polished and they end up useless."

~ Chris Colfer

Chapter 17

Detoxification of the Soul Body

"Diseases of the soul are more dangerous and more numerous than those of the body."
~ Cicero

When it comes to the soul body, although its causes, effects and remedies vastly resemble that of the emotional body, we are dealing with a mostly abstract concept which falls under the category of metaphysics. The soul body is considered to be an etheric, invisible, and impalpable level of the body. Metaphysical scholars have said that the soul is encoded with a large amount of information about our life's purpose and evolutionary status. The soul has an agenda pertaining to its evolution. Human thinking and behaviors are a reflection of universal consciousness. The soul carries imprints of frequencies from different levels of consciousness.

Carl Jung has written: *"I simply believe that some part of the human Self or Soul is not subject to the laws of space and time."*

For millennia, wise Indigenous cultures from all five continents have posited that:

> Every soul is on a mission but some souls have been derailed from their course. Some other souls are roaming around looking for something that they cannot find and they dwell in a state of despair. Whatever condition the soul is in, it is related to a person's life path. Some souls are here to accomplish a set purpose, whether they are on a very quick or a very long journey.

> The soul has a memory. It holds encodings of data amounting to the sum total of all sorts of experiences stored for eons of time or in different dimensions of time. Researchers who are familiar with quantum physics or quantum mechanics are familiar with this concept that may seem arcane or obscure to the average mind.

> Souls also face the challenge of having to balance specific traits from the ego with the difficulties of living in the physical realm. A lot of the challenges the soul faces has to do with a reintegration process. Through such process, one has to learn how to survive or evolve while reconciling encoded cellular memory with the necessity of mastering a new physical environment. The soul, just as the physical body necessitates detoxification.

Each indigenous tradition has its own set of practitioners that are trained to identify and bring remedies to issues pertaining to the soul. Usually, the practitioners who handle affairs pertaining to the soul are secular or non-secular priests and priestesses, shamans, medicine men/women, etc. The said practitioners are trained disciplines pertaining to esoteric or metaphysical practices. On all five continents, there are shamans in many types of traditions, some of which are: Native American, South American, African, Druidistic, Hawaiian, Huna, Kahuna, Siberian, Buddhist, etc. Being an authentic shaman involves devoting one's life and energies to healing other people from conditions that are not otherwise detected or understood by other modern, conventional, high technology, left brain oriented cultures.

Regardless of the tradition, basically all shamanic practitioners agree that soul issues usually stem from an original wound. Quite often, the original wound relates to abuse, neglect, rape, abandonment, accidents, and any other type of physical or psychological trauma. If not addressed or healed soon after its occurrence, this wound gets carried throughout life and causes an unending chain of difficulties for the wounded person. Detoxification helps heal from trauma at the level of the psyche.

"Good humor is the health of the soul; sadness is its poison"

~ Lord Chesterfield

Alberto Villoldo, Ph.D., a psychologist and anthropologist who has trained in the Inca shamanic healing tradition for more than 25 years also trains individuals as practitioners of energy therapy. Shamanic practitioners understand that the soul or part of it can be lost. The soul is that part of the body that is infinite. Dr. Villoldo teaches that after a traumatic event, a part of the human energy field called the luminous body usually ends up being damaged. He suggests that healing the luminous body is very important if one is to experience recovery on all levels of the person.

Trauma always has detrimental repercussions on the physical and mental bodies. It is a fact that people who have survived domestic violence, long-term family drama, combat, serious vehicular accidents, major surgery, and any other type of major psychological shock usually end up expressing soul fragmentation and soul loss, which in Western psychiatry is labeled as Post Traumatic Stress Disorder (PTSD) a condition that carries the same symptoms as soul loss. In all cases, the psychological trauma that someone endures usually translates into a high level of toxicity to the person's body and mind. Unless the psychological body is detoxified from trauma, the physical body may not heal.

Moreover, ancient Indigenous traditions indicate that:
> In traditional Indigenous medicine, the soul is recognized as an essential part of the self that directly influences the states of health or dis-ease for the mind or body. There are various degrees in which the soul can be damaged through the experience of trauma. The damage can range from fragmentation to total soul loss. In many people, this damage is experienced in the form of chronic illnesses that may appear to be psychosomatic and are not always detectable through conventional tests. In other cases, the soul loss can manifest itself in the form of terminal illnesses and oftentimes physical death. A lot of the

time, the aspects of the soul's ills are directly related to toxicity. Because the soul can be affected by toxicity, it is therefore important to become knowledgeable on the subject matter if one is to seriously know how to detoxify the self on all possible levels.

The knowledge of soul healing, has been orally transmitted to chosen people from various indigenous cultures. Natives usually are more apt at understanding the process of soul damage compared to others who are neither exposed to the culture nor privy to secrets of ancient traditions. Such secrets were usually reserved to royalty and high-ranking members of the clergy who have been privy to carefully preserved knowledge for generations. A huge body of secret ancient knowledge relates to the invisible part of the person called the soul.

Almost fifty percent of Americans experience depression and are on anti-depressants. Oftentimes, people stay on such medications for years. Based on this fact, it appears that it is time that people look at their issues from a different angle than the mere physical one. It is easy to deny or discount evidence that is not visible to the naked eye, and that mechanical testing is not capable of evaluating. Indigenous sages say that there are other issues that pertain to the soul which are not simply in the domain of the physical, mental, or emotional bodies. For example, some people are not comfortable being of a particular gender or being locked into a particular gender role. Sages also explain that in some cases, parents were hoping for a male baby but ended up disappointed with the birth of a baby girl. In other cases, the soul of a female accommodates a male body without expectations from the parents. On many levels, various issues with the soul are passed down at the DNA level from one generation to another, and often for several generations. Soul program issues are complex.

In many ways, the soul can act a lot like the physical body when under stress. This explains why the soul is subjected to the fight-or-flight dynamic. When under the leash of traumatic circumstances, the soul can either become fragmented or choose to take flight, depending on the degree of severity of the circumstance. Soul fragmentation is responsible for physical and psychological conditions that usually do not have a remedy in physical treatments. In some cases of trauma, it may not be possible for certain individuals to humanly handle the level of pain or shock that the trauma entails. Consequently, their soul may choose to manage the situation by fragmenting itself and allowing the fragments to take flight from the body. In some extreme cases, once departed from the body, the soul fragments may choose not to return. Skilled shamans are capable of going to an immaterial space called the underworld to negotiate with souls for the return of their fragments. Reintegration depends on the cases and the level of toxicity or trauma that has damaged the soul. Besides soul fragmentation, damage to the soul can extend itself to soul loss. Most known soul healing processes comprise clearing the soul from the energetic frequency of trauma, through detoxifying methods.

"The soul, like the body, lives by what it feeds on."

~ Josiah Gilbert Holland

To a spiritually untrained person, the signs of soul loss may not be understood. Untrained or unaware people may argue that the unseen is either absurd or unscientific, therefore is to be dismissed. It is this very type of bias that may indicate signs of soul loss or pineal gland deterioration or calcification in such people. Soul loss and pineal gland calcification are known for dulling the sixth sense.

Some signs of soul fragmentation and soul loss are as follows:

- Depression symptoms including suicidal impulses, deep sadness, and despair.
- Personality changes such as apathetic behavior and isolationism.
- Sudden emotional detachment.
- Disorientation.
- Inability to feel or express genuine emotions.
- Chronic self-sabotage.
- Memory issues.
- Lack of touch with reality, spaciness, brain fog, dementia and delirium symptoms.
- Dullness of the senses / decrease of natural instincts.
- Addictions to alcohol, drugs, sexual promiscuity, vice, etc.
- Lack of motivation and drive in carrying life's obligations and duties.
- Disconnection from source energy.
- Inability to understand energetic dynamics.

The remedies that traditional Indigenous shamans usually recommend for soul detoxification are:

Energetic Soul Clearing

This native treatment utilizes energy medicine methods associated with the use of healing plants and flowers, sound frequencies, drum beats, vision quest, minerals, stones, and re-connecting to Earth. The basis of this clearing is energetic detoxification for cellular regeneration.

Soul Retrieval

It is a re-framing process in which the person is encouraged to take a mental journey to find and heal their soul's fragments, constructively re-writing a new script and overriding the past.

Soul Extraction

It involves extruding toxic emotions from the soul, clearing it from the trauma that has affected it, then re-calibrating the soul for its reintegration into active life with renewed resilience.

For levity:

"I was thrown out of college for cheating on the
metaphysics exam: I looked into the soul of another boy."

~ Woody Allen

Chapter 18

Detoxification from Toxic People

"You have the right to quit toxic people. They are contagious."
~ Dr. Sun Wolf

As long as there are toxic people living on the planet, there will be conflict. Because of the very nature of the interconnectedness of all people, it is unrealistic and even counterproductive to seek to live in complete isolation just to avoid toxic individuals. Toxic people carry the essence of conflict. They are experts at finding their prey so they can create artificial conflicts in order to meet their narcissistic agenda. The main construct of toxic people is to initiate conflict where there is none because that is what validates their existence. There are numerous causes for emotional toxicity; they range from neurotoxins that cause depression to genetic defects.

It is the wide spectrum of differences among the members of the collective that makes it difficult to consistently be in harmony. The duality game translates into conflicting thoughts and opinions, attitudes and determinations of fate. Some people want to abuse all power and enslave others. Some play gods and take the lives of others on a whim if they feel that their ego is threatened in one way or another. Most murder victims – about 60% – are killed by people they know, and oftentimes, within their household. Our world is filled with dangerous, impatient, mentally unstable, violent, and out of control people. The constant in all of them is fear.

Individuals who were born and raised in abusive families or institutions may be habituated to the abuse to the point of being unable to see the good in others. They are obsessed with projecting it onto others. Because toxic abuse is the only model such people know, they do not have any other frame of reference to compare their abusiveness to. The only model they have to compare their abusiveness to is the abuse itself. As a result, they remain stuck in an ongoing pattern of abuse. Such people treat people around them abusively, mistreat their own family members, mates, friends, co-workers, and abuse their own self. Obnoxious people are usually affected by intestinal toxicity that is energetically affecting their brain and their thought processes, therefore their energetic output. They often are very constipated people, suffering from toxemia, therefore processing colon, liver, and kidney diseases such as cancer. Many of these people compound their toxicity with an addiction to recreational drugs, alcohol, tobacco, or pharmaceutical drugs.

Different types of toxic people

1. **The judge:** they make their point by criticizing in a destructive, rather than a constructive way. They enjoy being condescending or irreverent, using tactics such as blaming and reprimanding. They feel secure when they think you are under their control. They often experience a high rate of addiction and depression, and also gallbladder and liver issues.

2. **The imposter:** they first present themselves as polite, caring, concerned people, full of promises and integrity, wanting to sell you their business services. Then when it comes to acting upon their promises, after they get your money, they make an about face and immediately turn harsh, disrespectful, do not pick up the phone or pick-up just to tell you that they will call back but never do. They usually are liars, thieves, and chronic addicts.

3. **The excuse-maker:** they are shamelessly irresponsible people capable of developing very elaborate excuses to cover up their unreliability. They are always going through a major drama in their life. They usually end up dishonoring you with their lack of integrity. The bottom line is their issues with commitment phobia and lack of self-respect.

4. **The control freak:** they are mostly narcissists who are master manipulators and feel that they have to exercise control over you by any means, usually through sabotage. Their tactics work in such a way that when they know your timeline, they sabotage your deadline; if they know your needs, they ignore them or trick you with broken promises. They ensure that your need is not met; if they know your weaknesses they perversely make it sound like you are foolish in the way you handle your challenges; if they do something that resembles a favor to you, they ensure that it is mostly to their advantage; they may also use reproach and vilify or exploit you in condescending ways.

5. **The abuser:** they may be well behaved for a while, then soon turn abusive, particularly if they are under the influence of drugs or alcohol. The abuse is usually verbal before it turns physical. Someone who is verbally abusive is also prone to physical abuse. They may become irrational when challenged and end up harming their loved ones. Most abusers are dangerous narcissists. They usually have liver and kidney issues.

6. **The parasite:** they are energy leaches that cannot have enough of you, your resources, and your time. They call you at odd hours and always have a problem that only you can solve. They expect you to rescue them daily and the favors you do are not only quickly forgotten but never returned. There is no such thing as an equal exchange with a parasite. They may be plagued by different kinds of intestinal parasites due to internal toxicity.

7. **The amnesiac:** they make promises that they do not and cannot keep. They either wax apologetic when you remind them of their promise or blow up in anger stating that they never said or promised anything. They are disorganized people lacking self-governance.

8. **The envy:** whatever you have, they want, whether it is your mate, your car, your home, your looks, your success, etc. They feel pain when something good is in the offing for you. They covertly connive and covertly rain on your parade. They relish distorting your character and may insinuate false flaws or weaknesses about you, just to boost their ego.

9. **The naysayer:** they usually discount your values and accomplishments. They feel good making you feel small and insignificant. They trivialize your projects and may voice that the good things you are expecting 'cannot happen and must not happen'. These people have the most self- sabotage issues who also have significant anger stored in their liver.

10. **The cheat:** they are disloyal, flirting in your face and cheating behind your back. Lying and conniving also come with their cheating. They may cheat on a good mate mostly because their insecurity causes them to secure backup. They do cheat because they simply have a weak and disloyal nature. They often end up having heart and kidney issues.

11. **The bully:** they always have to be right. They do not have their act together, but because they are unruly rebels with major self-hatred and guilt, they abuse other people who may call them on their dysfunctional behaviors. Their seemingly tough behavior is just a cover-up for their fragile, easily wounded core. They have a hard time handling pain so once they are wounded, they lock themselves into a hard-as-steel shell, hoping that their toughness will prevent future wounds. They often have liver, heart, and kidney issues.

12. **The gossip:** they always have the latest story to tell you about someone else's private life, even if you do not have any kind of relationship with the person. Conversely, they feel compelled to disclose your private life to others too. Other people's life is their main form of entertainment because theirs is boring. These are people with a deep sense of void in their life. They enjoy exposing others in an attempt to make their shortcomings look pale or inexistent in comparison to those of other people. They may have spleen and heart issues.

Due to the multi-dimensionality of people's character, the above types are not to be misconstrued as compartmentalized. The character types may be found combined in a lot of individuals, with an exhibition of a few or all of the above-mentioned traits. The complexity of people's character causes them to display some traits more than others, depending on the circumstances.

*All violent feelings produce in us a falseness in all our impressions of external
things, which I would generally characterize as the "Pathetic Fallacy."*

~ John Ruskin

Those who resemble assemble. Due to different levels of affinities, there is always an energetic reason why people come together, even in cases where opposites seem to attract. It is in your best interest to assess the pros and cons of maintaining a relationship with a toxic person. Due to frequency exchanges when someone's negativity is overwhelming, it can energetically contaminate the less toxic person who comes into contact with the more toxic one. It is not unusual to see someone start mimicking the behavior of someone else they have frequent interaction with. Someone's manner of speaking, eating habits, and lifestyle, can all be modified when someone consciously or unconsciously chooses to adapt to some other person's way of being; if the lifestyle is toxic, the negative influence is a detriment.

Action steps for energetic detoxification from a toxic person's negativity

1. Do self-evaluation and look for insights on energetic causes and effects.

2.   Determine to uncover what underlying or hidden causes exist in you, and what causes the person to echo them to you. Because we are all mirrors of each other, whether we want to hear it or not, we unconsciously reflect behaviors. Each person is in our life to show us what needs correction within us. Once the correction is effected, then there is no more need for us to act as energetic reflectors. Be aware that this is not an instant process.

3. Confront the toxic person if you feel the emotional strength to do so, and do it compassionately. Let them know how you feel when they act in toxic ways. Suggest they seek professional help. Meet on neutral grounds and in public, to ensure that you are safe in their presence at that time.

4.   Do not position yourself in a victim's role because it is a dis-empowering perception that gives the toxic person leverage over you.

5.   Make a conscious decision to change the pattern of abuse by changing yourself and your attitude toward them.

6. Take some time to disconnect and let go of resentment toward the toxic person.

7. Take the time to analyze their strategies based on past behavior that usually predicts future moves.

8. Practice Ho'Oponopono and sincerely wish them well.

9. Practice Emotional Freedom Technique (EFT).

10. Keep healthier boundaries in the future.

For levity:

"Men are beasts, and even beasts don't behave as they do."

~ Brigitte Bardot

Chapter 19

Detoxification from Toxic Relationships

"One is better off alone in dignity rather than in a relationship that demands a sacrifice of one's self-respect ."

~ Anon

Countless people initiate personal relationships because of what they believe is love. Among all things, love is the best reason for entering into relationships but it is also the most misinterpreted.

What is love?

Unlike what most people think, love is neither a feeling, nor a strong reaction to visceral emotions that may simply be related to possessiveness, jealousy, and lust. Love is an attitude of benevolence and compassion, the resultant of the qualities of patience, kindness, humility, and respect. Loving is to rise above the pettiness of illusions from emotions. The ability to exercise and practice love versus reactions in the face of flip-flopping energies is what separates the men from the boys and the women from the girls. When you are big enough in personality to ensure that even those who feel that they have to be your worst enemies are treated compassionately, then you are operating at the level of avatars and Zen masters. It is not the emotions we feel that count, but the mastery we have over the said emotions. If more humans were capable of reaching this level of self-mastery, there would be fewer crimes of passion and less envy.

Love is patient, love is kind. It does not envy or boast;
it is not arrogant.

~ 1 Corinthians 13:4

Development of a toxic relationship

To the person under the mesmerization of seduction, it may take a while to detect a toxic relationship. For the most part, people pay attention enough to be on their best behavior at the beginning of a relationship. The more eager to ensnare they are, the more pleasing they behave.

Soon, however, the veneer of pleasantness disappears and the beast turns loose. It may take just a comment that the toxic person perceives as threatening to make their veneer crack or chip, exposing the other layers of personality that are underneath. What makes the relationship toxic is the pathology of one or both partners. Because of vibrational frequency matches, there usually is a commonality that contains a life lesson which has caused the attraction in the first place. In general, there is an energetic commonality that attracts toxic people to us and vice versa.

Many toxic relationships come with one partner that is more toxic than the other. This particular partner is usually a toxic time bomb. The toxic time bomb may start by doing good things for you to create goodwill and earn your trust and confidence. While you relax about being in a relationship with whomever you perceive to be a good person, subversive activity may have already started; usually, this is the beginning of the end.

Red flags to watch for

1. Emotional unavailability
In a toxic relationship, partners are often mismatched. In many cases one of them is not emotionally available mostly because they are already tied to someone else emotionally or legally, and they are unhappy in that relationship too. In many situations, there are older people who are not ready for a relationship but seek the benefits of non-committal companionship with someone else in case of a divorce or separation. Some people may engage in helicopter parenting, a behavior that causes them to over-parent through excessive involvement in, and control over, their adult children's lives. This allows the person to resist full emotional involvement with you by focusing on their grown offspring. Often, people seek to avoid maintaining or building a relationship with a new mate mostly because their expectations of life-long mating have been violated through divorce or separation. Unfortunately, helicopter parenting inhibits their young adults' resourcefulness while impeding their coping and survival skills.

2. Misplaced priorities
In a toxic relationship, people's priorities can be grotesquely misplaced. They may put emphasis on maintaining an addiction to drugs or alcohol, illicit sex, etc. They may neglect basic needs for food, shelter, personal care, education, savings, etc. At times, the indulgent person might not be able to make the distinction between a luxury and a necessity. Often this situation takes a toll on the less toxic partner's emotions. The toxic partner is often in a financial predicament mostly because self-indulgence is their priority.

3. The ongoing seduction of the promise

A toxic person may manipulate their way into acceptance by offering a better carrot than anyone else around. Although the person may not be in a financial or personal situation to fulfill certain promises, they insist on making unrealistic promises they know they cannot keep.   In fact, there is no real effort put into fulfilling the promise. It is designed to monopolize the other person's attention and keep playing the seduction game.

4. Your world revolves around the other person's

You end up often changing your schedule, lifestyle, and healthier habits not necessarily because it is your choice but because the toxic partner has major needs that always appear more important than yours.   A lot of the time, choices are made for you before you are even informed of them. Your terms are likely to be disputed or dismissed. Even when you are asked about your preferences, you still find yourself being convinced that the partner's way is the better way. Watch the subtleties when you are invited for a meal in a restaurant. Things are conducted in accordance with the other person's preferences.

5. Endless bait and switch

You are asked to do certain things for the party but once you agree, you end up being asked to accommodate them in other ways. You may have to deal with a lot of hidden agenda. Usually, the other party makes the switch in a way that may dis-empower or disrespect you. You may think you have some form of covenant with the person, but the next thing you know is that they are conning you.

6. There is no real interaction with you or attention to you

You may notice the person's obvious inattentiveness toward you. There may be little eye contact. The inattentiveness toward you is a form of passive aggression disguised as busy mode, just to shut you out. You may end up feeling as if you are an inconvenience to the person, but only an accessory to them until they have the next urge to merge. Their behavior may prevail particularly in cases where the person lacks integrity toward you and knows it. When the person shuts you out of their attentiveness, it is to prevent you from having the opportunity to express yourself. They know that your self-expression could put them on the spot and expose them.

7. Cheating

Any action or intention relating to a sexual exchange of energy with a third party when one is in a relationship with someone else constitutes cheating. The act of cheating can be: physical, covert, overt, or emotional. On any level, cheating is particularly difficult to handle when the non-cheating partner is caring and devoted. Even some of the most devoted partners may unconsciously contribute to the cheating if they are not able to meet all of their partner's needs -- especially when the partner's needs are excessive.

In most cases, the cheating partner lies to the other. When this happens, the cheating partner's lack of disclosure additionally violates the other partner's right to make an informed choice to move on or seek to remedy the situation.

Cheating is one of the most major reasons why people split. If a toxic mate's energy is with other people while they are in a relationship with you, they are not energetically devoted to you. Not only they are emotionally scattered, but also they are energetically unclean. The uncleanliness can lead to disease transmission and energetic cross-contamination. Cheating usually tends to be a recurrent behavior; so once a cheat, always a cheat.

In either overt or covert emotional cheating, the person may be very obsessed with someone else to the point that even though they are not having a physical affair, they are addicted to each other. They are always arranging to meet behind your back and sometimes, even in your face! Sometimes, you may even be called by the other person's name, which reveals where the toxic partner's focus is. There may be transference of energies to the point that the cheating partner may use their memory of the other person's affection to feel tantalized while with you, and make you believe that it is you that they desire. At times, cheats require a smoke screen as a decoy to cover up their operations. They may set up special ringtones on their phones or establish hidden folders in their computer. They may compulsively delete every email, text or phone number that may reveal their activity. Some cheats may use domestic violence when caught, in an effort to gain control over their situation.

8. Measuring

The toxic person may put other people before you and even state that they love or care for the other people more than you. It may be a business partner or their family members. This indicates a contrived sense of measurement as well as a lack of tact and personal maturity. When someone loves you in a selfless way, they do not make it sound like others are more important than you. Any effort to quantify or measure love by establishing that you are the less important recipient of their attention is a standard that clearly shows an avoidance of commitment. Where there is sincere love, it is equitably distributed without being contemptuously gauged.

9. Your needs are ignored, left unmet, or dismissed.

This is a sign that selfishness, immaturity, and disrespect prevail on the other party's side. You may also experience the degradation of not having your desires and needs taken seriously. For instance, you may have scheduled to spend time with the person and they were in agreement with you at the time. Later, the arrangement may be canceled to the benefit of some business meeting or personal escapade. When this happens on a regular basis, it is a signal that your needs for a human connection do not matter to the person. In case the need is emotional, the person may have emotional blocks associated with past trauma. The blocks may prevent the person from interacting with another through normal empathy, closeness, or affection. It usually is a sign of resentment toward you.

10. Denial

The party may have memory issues due to brain damage caused by drugs or alcohol abuse to the point of blacking out. They make statements, plans, or promises that they can no longer remember. When faced with the issue, instead of considering that they may have a problem, they instead proceed to vehemently deny saying anything. Usually, denial is a conclusive sign confirming the existence of amnesia, convenient or not.

11. Major friction when you call the person on their lack of self-governance
This denotes un-coachability and conceit. No one is perfect and we can all use some objective awareness from others. When you call someone on their faulty behavior and you do it in a compassionate and non-offensive way, if they overreact, it indicates an ego issue that makes them stuck. This type of person is not going to learn from their shortcomings. What you say may expose a deficiency in the individual's personality. If they interpret your words as button-pushing rather than an opportunity to correct their dysfunction, then the person is not ready to face their impediment in a mature way. The individual is in the way of their own their self-growth. If they attack you and shift blame, then they are dealing with major countertransference issues.

12. Inflexibility
If everything is always the person's way or no way, their tyranny indicates emotional issues with control. There is often an *'either or'* clause to everything they do with you. If they do not respect your wisdom, wishes, or schedule, they do not respect you.

The role of emotional issues in toxic relationships

A mentally or emotionally imbalanced person who is unable to function normally within a relationship may be suffering from Post Traumatic Stress Disorder (PTSD) from child abuse, rape, exposure to domestic violence, combat, substance abuse, etc. They may also be affected by parasitism, candidiasis, and chemical imbalances. If they are aware of their ordeal, there may be hope for them provided that they are willing to commit to treatment. If not, there is not much that love can do to remedy a situation in which a person might be too damaged to be functional. Most of the symptoms of PTSD-related dysfunction are:

- Extreme agitation, unexplainable irritability, impatience, and self-control issues.
- Sleeplessness, night terrors, torment due to flashbacks, etc.
- Inability to relax / Hypervigilance / Hyperarousal.
- Difficulty focusing and a constant need to multi-task.
- Self image insecurity.
- Self-hating, self-denying, and self-destructive behavior / Erratic behavior.
- Compulsive overeating / Emotional eating often triggered by stressors.
- Addictions: compulsive drinking and / or drug abuse.
- Memory loss issues / Inability to process and retain new information.
- Weight issues.
- Refusal to talk about the trauma / A need to shut down / Isolationism.
- Avoidance of meaningful relationships and focus on self-distraction.
- Compulsive masturbation that may be enjoyed more than love-making.
- Compulsive need for controlling other people, things, or situations.
- Reckless handling of one's personal, business affairs, and relationships.
- Extreme disorganization.
- Ineffectiveness in daily affairs.
- Chronic refusal to accept help.
- Oppositional defiance.

It is not always easy to determine what to do about our relationship because besides other issues, such relationship may involve deep emotional attachments. Many people say that they follow their heart and choose to remain in a relationship with a conflict-prone mate because they simply feel that they cannot live without the person. Others say that they continue to be part of a conflict-habituated relationship with someone for their learning experience. In this case, they use their love to weather the storm of the other person's abusiveness. The effective management of conflicts can provide them with the human skills they need to understand their life's purpose.

Individuals with self-hatred issues are not going to engage in harmonious relationships with anyone, regardless of how much they are loved. They cannot give what they do not have. Some people are chronically harsh with others. This type of person has issues with major liver toxicity. When you have to deal with frequent power struggles with someone who has no regard for your feelings, it is a sign that you must seek therapeutic intervention. If that fails, you require taking time out and clear your own energies from the person's toxicity and your own.

It is important to understand that we attract in our lives people who are a vibrational match to us. If we are able to unconsciously attract certain entities in our energy field, it is also our prerogative to heal ourselves from the traits we have in common with them. For us to stop vibrating with people we feel no longer have anything in common with us, it is important to change our outlook on what the relationship means to us. It is important to be thankful for the lessons the person has come into our lives to teach us. People can free themselves from the dysfunction when they are aware of their patterns. At times, being free from a dysfunctional relationship is healthier than remaining a slave to it. People who are aware of their own faulty relational template have an emotional advantage over those who are not aware of it. The awareness itself maximizes the power to rectify the dysfunctional template.

Negative patterns and misunderstanding

Otentimes, even when people make an honest effort to find remedies to a toxic situation, a pattern of self-sabotage may ensue. The self-sabotage is very likely to manifest itself through counterproductive postponement or delays that undermine all efforts to resolve the issue.
The reasons for this usually are:

- People get stuck in patterns of self-doubt, passive aggression, and more.
- Society trains people to be more automaton-like than human-like.
- When their ego is imbalanced, some individuals may feel attacked if they are exposed to a more constructive way to function.
- Most people feel that their identity is threatened with loss.
- Often, a person's efforts to resolve their pattern issues are unproductive if they approach a solution at the conscious level instead of subconsciously.
- Change takes work and it is scary to those who are not ready for it. People may feel that they are not capable of handling the inconveniences of change.
- Some dysfunctional people are attached to their negative pattern, particularly if this is all they are used to. That is one of the many reasons why countless survivors of abuse defend their abuser(s).

Reasons for loving the self

To love others, you first have to love yourself. Humans treat the world as they treat themselves. If you treat yourself like a junkyard dog, or an abandoned clunker parked in the ghetto's empty lot, you will do the same to others, even to those who love you the most. Some people treat their cars better than themselves. They do an oil change, car wash, polish, and interior vacuuming; but when it comes to their own person, oftentimes there is no incentive to be self-nurturing. Yet, these toxic people desire to be in a relationship. When things go bad, it does not occur to the affected individuals that it is time to make an effort and look at themselves. Most humans look for people, things, or situations to put the blame on. They avoid taking responsibility for the situations they create. The mirror effect causes us to have the 'benefit' of having other people reflect back to us what requires healing in ourselves. It is always very important to acknowledge what we see in another person as a wake up call. At times, it is an unmistakable indication of what needs to be addressed within us for our own recovery from childhood disempowerment.

Unconditional love and acceptance contribute to demonstrating that you are – emotionally and spiritually – more mature than a toxic narcissist who persists in battling or challenging you. You can advocate for their healing and rehabilitation by exercising compassion over them, just like a loving parent would do for their rebellious two year old in the middle of a temper tantrum. Remember that narcissists are mostly people who have unresolved childhood trauma and have the additional disadvantage of being stuck in a specific pattern of dysfunction. They feel trapped in the pattern and that makes them regress to the age they were when they experienced the trauma, acting immaturely because they are stuck. Contrary to popular belief, narcissists do not love themselves. They create an illusion of self-love through sustained ego gratification to counteract the self-loathing that they are battling within, or the shame and guilt they are hiding.

Reasons for accepting the self

Over time, when one accepts the self, the barriers that have existed between unloving, toxic people and us may either fall or close permanently. As people are like mirrors, reflecting back to us, what we must face in order to address our hidden issues, when we receive their message, we must do it in humility and gratitude if we are to heal. When we learn to accept that even though we are not perfect we must keep doing the best we can, then it is easier for us to evolve. If we are true to our self, our subconscious will re-arrange the circumstances in our lives. This might entail seeing a more accepting picture of ourselves through others. Consequently, the rejection and harshness we experienced through toxic people may change their configuration as we heal.

Reasons for forgiving

Forgiveness is not only to the benefit of the toxic people who offend us but also for ours. When we release pain projected onto us and forgive a toxic person, we also release ourselves from negative energetic implications. This only can protect us from illnesses, many of which are due to processing toxic emotions that may change the blood's pH and make it more acidic than necessary. Hyperacidity usually leads to toxicity, disease, and death. It is scientifically proven that cancer, diabetes, and arthritis are symptoms deriving from an inability to forgive and move on.

The more steadfast you stand in your ability to be bigger than the pain you feel during your challenge, the more skilled you become at managing your situation. Being flexible also counts but that does not mean cannot be firm. Just remember to ensure that equity prevails. Detachment is healing for people whose frequencies do not match. When you love and accept yourself, it is easier for you to not take so personally what toxic people make happen for you. By the power of the law of cause-and-effect, and by the power of the law of return, what others make happen for you, they bring upon themselves. The whole matter may have its basis in psychological warfare. Even though it may have its roots in causes that the average mind cannot understand, unforgiveness is not only a waste of your time but also a self-defeating proposition.

"Forgiveness doesn't always lead to a healed relationship.
Some people are just not capable of love and it might be wise
to let them go, along with your anger. Just wish them well
and take care of yourself."

~ Anon

Beyond forgiveness

In some cases, forgiveness is not enough to mend a toxic relationship. Due to childhood issues, some men are very angry at women and some women very angry at men: these toxic individuals are very hard to heal. Gender-based anger is one of the reasons why pornography is so successful: it provides the toxic person with the form of sublimation they seek to degrade another person. When forgiveness is not what it takes, one has to learn to let go. Some toxic people are not only unloving but also unlovable. They are damaged beyond repair. They can neither love nor desire to love. Toxic people do not want to learn how to love because that is not their priority. When you let go of someone who is a toxic time bomb, then you may discover a being who is loving and lovable – you -- if that is truly what you are. When you discover the loving person that you may be, you are re-empowered. Learn to free-flow and let go! As you release yourself from the self-imposed obligation to love an unlovable toxic being, you learn to love yourself for what you are. It frees you up to attract a vibrational match, if that is your goal.

It is a false sense of responsibility to insist on working on toxic people's salvation if they are adamant that they do not want to upgrade or change. When they lash out at you, keep your feelings in check and get them under control as soon as possible. Remember that you have the power to be in control of your emotions, if you are self-governed. It is those who are slaves to their emotions that allow lack of control to rule and manipulate them. It is really hard to be truly magnanimous when dealing with a chronically toxic mate; when the toxic person is verbally and physically abusive, lying, cheating, stealing, conniving and expressing sheer irresponsibility and hostility, we must keep practicing forgiveness. We must also learn to release and let go of what is injurious to our dignity, self-esteem, and sanity. To the measure of our spiritual strength, our desire to heal relates to our decision to forgive and move on. It is essential that we explore our courage and expand it to the measure of our capabilities for higher understanding of what to do.

142

Useful therapies for detoxification from toxic relationship issues:

Deep breathing, cleansing, and clearing exercises

Example: Imagine the hurt in your heart as having a shape. Identify its location, color, and size. Now tell the part of yourself that has been holding onto the hurt that it is time to let it go. Open the mouth and slowly breathe out the hurt. Imagine the hurt dissolving in red light. Then take a deep inhalation through the nose, imagining you are breathing in white light. Hold the breath and imagine any residue of the hurt being cleansed and breathe out through the mouth. Then repeat the same process for the dissolution of any holographic representation of the hurt.

Hypnotherapy

It can be therapeutic on many levels, from stress relief to healthy detachment. As a therapeutic modality, hypnotherapy uses deep relaxation for the purpose of preparing the subject's mind to receive specific suggestions. A hypnotherapist may use various tones of voice that create different types of modulation and a range of relaxing frequencies ranging from alpha to gamma. By relaxing, a person enters a receptive mode in order to process beneficial suggestions usually intended to accomplish a particular goal. One can utilize the services of a trained hypnotherapist or learn self-hypnosis. This is not for individuals who have been diagnosed with mental disorders. One can learn self-hypnosis or explore it with the help of recordings targeting a specific purpose.

Hypnotherapy can also assist you in shifting your focus of attention from a toxic person to a productive goal in your life. If the toxic person's memory recurs in your thoughts, do repeat the hypnotherapy session until it is fully effective.

Another benefit of Hypnotherapy is its usefulness as a tool for healthy detachment from recurrent toxic thoughts. It can be used to blur, fade, edit, or delete your memory of a toxic experience for the purpose of lessening the burden of painful recall or flashback.

Ho'Oponopono

It is a very popular Hawaiian self-healing method based on forgiveness and gratitude. It consists of repeating: *"I am sorry, please forgive me, thank you, I love you."* as often as possible. Repeat until cathartic relief or neutral detachment occurs.

Mental detachment

It allows you to avoid being controlled by your own weakness, emotions, and the toxic person's negative vibrations. Remember that you are no longer a toxic vibrational match. Emotional detachment takes mental discipline and an elevated view of a situation. Allow yourself to use objectivity, reason, and compassion to look at the painful situation from a constructive angle. When you choose not to let pain be a dominant factor, you are more able to keep a clear agenda to be detached with civility and compassion in the best interest of all. Most humans act overly combative in the face of a necessity to detach from an emotionally toxic person or from a toxic situation. Choose to shift this toxic paradigm.

Emotional Freedom Technique

It is useful in reframing and reorganizing perceptions. Here is a sample exercise:

EFT for Healing the Pain of Toxic Relationships

Karate chop point: "Even though I feel that I am being provoked, disrespected, and dishonored by ___________ in this relationship, I choose to love and respect myself nevertheless."

Inner corner of the eye: "Even though at times – and especially now – I find the situation unbearable, I choose to realize that I have no choice but to initiate a change in my own attitudes now, in order to preserve my sanity."

Outer corner of the eye: "Even though I feel deeply provoked, I also acknowledge that I may have also provoked ___________, in one way or another, consciously or unconsciously. Therefore I choose to forgive myself and also choose to forgive ___________."

Under the eye: "Even though I may not always be conscious of ___________'s feelings, I choose to be more mindful of my actions from now on."

Under the nose: "Even though I feel angry at ___________ when he/she attacks, I choose to remember that I am the one who owns and controls my feelings. I also choose to understand the shame ___________ experiences when he/she perceives my communication as a judgment or an attack."

Chin: "Even though ___________ enjoys putting me to shame when attacking me, I choose to remember that I can teach him/her to treat me better by accepting, respecting and loving myself more."

Collar bone: "Even though I often feel like setting more boundaries to the point of terminating the relationship with ___________, I choose to remember to do that with respect and compassion nevertheless."

Armpit: "Even though ___________ is so harsh and disrespectful to me that I am tempted to seek revenge, I choose to see that he/she is conveying to me the message of something that needs to be addressed and healed within me."

Top of the head: "Even though I feel victimized in this relationship, I choose to take responsibility for the way I feel and be proactive rather than reactive. I choose to let go of oversensitivity and take my power back."

Heart: "Even though it is difficult to process the message that ___________ is mirroring to me, I choose to forgive him/her for the harshness of his communication and be grateful for the message. I choose to forgive myself for having created the condition within me for the lessons I must learn. I choose to be grateful to ___________ and the situation. And from now on, I love, respect, and accept myself totally and unconditionally."

It is useful to remember that when a vibrational mis-match is flagrant, any and all efforts to mend the relationship could be the equivalent of looking to fix broken glass. All you might end up with is bleeding cuts if you keep attempting such a worthless and perilous process. It is our attachments that usually cause sufferings. The fact that we are attached to toxic people indicates that we are to address our own toxicity first.

If there are indications that the mis-matched relationship is worthy of being salvaged, somehow, the lines of communications must be opened to clean the slate. Your own upgrade may rub-off on the other party over time and they may start refining their energies. If this does not occur, send the party good thoughts and wishes. From your heart, sincerely wish them happiness and leave it at that. You no longer need to dance with a toxic time bomb if you are the more aware of the two. Toxic people will either keep doing what they have been doing, expecting different results and experiencing their share of disappointment. They will keep entering and exiting toxic relationships with other toxic people who match their frequency, or they will start changing their ways if they have enough sense to begin detoxifying themselves.

Importance of the heart

The heart has its own autonomous nervous system and scientists say that the heart is smarter than the brain. Wilson Chilton-Pearce, author of *The Biology of Transcendence* refers to the heart as *"the major biological apparatus within us and the seat of our greatest intelligence."* Humans express love through the heart; love is capable of healing all types of situations at the levels of body, mind, spirit, and soul. The heart's love-based wisdom supersedes the brain's ego-based intelligence.

For levity:

As he lay on his deathbed, the man confided to his wife, "I cannot die without telling you the truth. I cheated on you throughout our whole marriage. All those nights when I told you I was working late, I was with other women. And not just one woman either, but I've slept with dozens of them."

His wife looked at him calmly and said, "I've always known it dear. Why do you think I poisoned you?"

~Anon

Chapter 20

Detoxification and Attitudes Adjustment

"Human beings, by changing the inner attitudes of their minds, can change the outer aspects of their lives."

~ William James

Complete and successful detoxification usually comes with noticeable attitudes adjustments that usually take place over time. What happens after your detoxification process has purified your energy field? You are likely to shift your energies to the point that obvious change starts occurring in your life. Change is likely to occur in the areas that one is the most ready for. For some people, change manifests itself in the domain of health; for others it happens with their relationships, whether personal or business; for others, change may appear in the domain of finances or personal growth. In certain people, all of the above can start shifting and aligning positively when their detoxified energies allow them to adjust and free flow. Change can range from subtle to significant, however the curve related to the change is not necessarily linear.

What you may experience as you shift

When your vibrational frequency changes, you shift your attitudes to a more constructive mode. You may start re-evaluating your priorities and see the meaningfulness or the meaninglessness of things in your life in a new light. You may start respecting yourself more to stop unproductive and harmful behaviors. You may hear people comment about how different you look now, how you look slimmer or younger, etc. When people around you energetically sense what is happening in you, eventually, they change their attitudes toward you accordingly. In general, other people reflect back to us the unconscious beliefs we have about ourselves.

Shift in relationships: once your energies have become purified and expanded, you are likely to start seeing a noticeable change in attitudes in the people in your life. When you are no longer a vibrational match to toxic people, a clearing occurs and people on either side start reaching a higher level of awareness that exposes flaws in a toxic relationship. You may start moving out of your comfort zone to explore other possibilities relating to the new frequencies you are vibrating with. You may feel that you no longer have to be another person's perpetual doormat. Individual reactions will depend on each party's level of evolution or toxicity.

Indicators of successful detoxification

The signs that the detoxification process is successful are as follows:

- The ability to uncover the foolishness and immaturity behind certain actions.
- Shedding extra weight more easily than before.
- Reduction or elimination of pain and other symptoms.
- Higher levels of energy.
- A new sense of freedom, joy, peace, or balance.
- Decreased irritability and anxiety.
- A new understanding of the true meaning of our connection with nature.
- The ability to relate to others with less fear.
- Experiencing more realistic expectations.
- The ability to forgive and move on.
- An ability to attract people who are a more harmonious vibrational match.
- Heightened awareness and intuition due to reconnection with source energy.
- More respect toward the body and the self.
- A deeper knowing that self-respect is more important than toxic relationships.

Possible reactions from other people about your shift

Usually, there are different voices that speak to us when we look to accomplish something meaningful. The voices can be as varied as the voice of completeness, the voice of doubt, and the voice of limitation.

1. **How people who are less toxic than you are likely to react**

   They are likely to start adjusting to your shift and feeling better around you, sensing that something has upgraded and they also, wish to be part of the experience. They are likely to be more pleasant to you and express the desire to be around you more. Some may ask you what it is that you are doing that feels different to them. They may feel inspired to also enhance their own life.

   Because life is a perpetual dance of energetic synchronization, it can be very uplifting when you have someone mirror your higher nature. This matching of frequencies usually shows you where you wish to be and with whom, in your decision to pursue a higher level of wellness. These people may start inviting you to go take a walk with them, or go explore some local venues for healthy activities. It can be releasing and encouraging to have your mirror reflect your highest potential.

How in-betweens are likely to react

Some people you encounter on your journey could be 'in-betweens'. They are exploring how to live a non-toxic life but their knowledge is not broad enough to afford them a solid conviction about the goodness of their exploration. In-betweens may be neutral toward you or may express doubt about the outcome of what you are doing.

How people who are more toxic than you are likely to react

When you start shifting into higher consciousness, you are no longer a vibrational match to the people from your pack, tribe or circle. Besides positive reactions from the first group described above, you might also see that other people may start acting suspicious of you. They may find you to be too different. For a lot of people, what is different is hard for them to analyze and understand, and is usually labeled as strange or threatening. So they may refer to you as a 'weirdo' or a 'freak'. They may say things like: *"Something strange is going on with Jane: now she won't go to the bar with us anymore, but she's drinking green stuff that looks like swamp water."* They are not quite exactly hostile but they are not quite accepting of you either. You are not quite exactly their opposite but you are not quite their vibrational match either. While these more toxic people are expressing a grade of non-constructive judgment toward you, their passive aggression may cause them to send you mixed signals. They cannot control their opinions because their need to judge you is bigger than themselves. There may be some expression of underlying anger or envy that you did not know existed in these toxic people. Their need to be right about their perceptions of you may inhibit their ability to see that they are the laggards in consciousness. While you are able to heal yourself, they are stuck in a spiral of illness, depression, addiction, helplessness, or an inability to shift.

Holding on to dysfunctions

When a person has their personality wrapped around their dysfunction, they may become so attached to it that it feels that they *are* their dysfunction. If it is the case that these individuals were born and raised in families that transmitted the same dysfunctional patterns from one generation to the other, then it is a very tough situation to bring remedies to. Some of the main stigmas people may hold on to are: depression, bigotry, racism, bad manners, ill eating habits, criminality, refusal to experience joy, etc.   Some individuals may have the opportunity to experience joy, however may not want to feel joyful if they are toxic. When people are guided more by their mis-qualified energies than by wisdom, it is a sign that the level of toxicity they operate with is pathological. Many humans choose illusions of comfort through unhealthy indulgences and addictions. Instead of bringing joy, these illusions cause toxic people to remain in a vicious cycle of conflict, self-hatred, and guilt. It is easy to get sidetracked and pulled into a different world of delusions, trickery, and deceit. Yet we are to remember who we truly are, even in the moments of most potent illusions. Some individuals are masters of illusions and are very skilled at pulling us in their world of tricks and deception. It happens for a specific learning experience: they are just doing their job as our life's teachers. The world is like a custom-made learning incubator: its lifelong nature never leaves us at a loss for opportunities to learn and grow.

It is a sad thing to see how toxic people prefer to put a claim on health issues and insist on referring to such issues as "theirs". For example, they speak of the issue, referring to their ills as: *"my cancer"*, *"my diabetes"*, *"my psoriasis"*, etc. A person may identify with the dysfunction so much that any mention of what may help with the issue is either dismissed or interpreted as an inconvenience. On some level, the person might need the dysfunction as a learning experience on their life's path. In some cases, encouraging them to let go of the dysfunction may even be an effort that can deprive them of an experience their soul may have chosen for its own evolution.

> *"Neurotics complain of their illness, but they make the most of it, and when it comes to taking it away from them they will defend it like a lioness defends her young."*
>
> ~ Sigmund Freud

Avoiding change

Sometimes you reach out to toxic people who are not responsive or receptive to the real lessons of life. When that happens, it usually comes with its share of pain and disappointments. Eventually, you have to realize that not only you are wasting your time, but you are also depriving yourself of valuable self-growth. What are you depriving yourself of? The interactive and constructive experience that may be available with other souls that are ready and willing to walk the path in harmony with you as your vibrational match. Usually the threat of death, surgery, imprisonment, and hell are the highest motivators for initiating change. When there is ill will and bad faith in someone, and when a situation brings you more pain than joy, you must courageously walk the other way. Your encouragement is not likely to be as strong as some life-threatening motivators.

You may sometimes make sensible recommendations that can make a difference to some toxic people but find out that these people express either apathy or resistance. You may find yourself repeating the same things until you are blue in the face without ever seeing a change in the toxic person's behavior. Quite often the person may claim that they have forgotten or may completely deny ever hearing what you have recommended. In this case, the matter has to do with a part of the person's psyche being so damaged that the damage may be irreversible and no amount of effort can help. The person may be a blackout drunk, an addict or genetically defective. Damage causes the person to be on a default setting, by way of a set program. The program is subconscious. Because the subconscious programs are very powerful, their default setting will keep overriding any new information. In case the toxic person is willing to change their situation, hypnosis can help. Without the desire to change, an issue cannot be effectively resolved.

Toxic people may find greater benefits in keeping their situation the way it is as opposed to changing it. Regardless of how dire the situation may appear to you and how unbearable the toxic person may claim it to be for them, they will not change. The benefits these toxic people perceive in their situation may outweigh the challenges of having to endure the inconvenience of shifting.

You can present beneficial ideas to toxic people but can never bring them to think. At times, you may show compelling evidence to someone about how changing their lifestyle from unhealthy to healthy would prolong their life, but they may not care. You may show them how upgrading their quality of life can allow them to start enjoying it more, they may still not care. In the event that they would be forced to change, they can also find a clever way to sabotage both the person encouraging them to change and their own self.

"Wisdom entereth not into a malicious mind."

~ Rabelais

The vibrational frequency of toxic individuals may not be high enough to allow them to uphold a certain level of wisdom and higher knowledge. They may therefore not be capable of properly interpreting a higher level of information as relevant to them. Even though the guidance may be timely and most appropriate for them at the moment, they may be too toxic to be able to resonate with subtle patterns. Since adjusting to new information takes effort and time, toxic people may feel inadequate or start believing that you are manipulating them. Instead of looking to understand new concepts by increment and grow through a search for meaning, they may fall into the usual mode of discrediting and sabotaging you for what their mind cannot process. As a result, toxic people may feel left out or initiate rejection. They may end up with a sense of frustration that is likely to have them start projecting anger or resistance toward you. Projection usually comes in ways that the toxic person proceeds to sabotage your life and theirs in the process. The sabotage process does not affect them so much because to them, sabotage is more the norm than the exception. In fact, the individuals will derive a sense of satisfaction from it because of the chaos it is likely to leave in its tracks. It is a fact that creating chaos can make toxic people feel more in control, thinking they have accomplished something.

Many toxic people thrive on chaos. That is one of the reasons why they replicate it wherever and whenever they can. Give them anything new and functional, orderly and organized, and they will trash it in no time and turn it into what they are most familiar and comfortable with: chaos. Usually, toxic people have such a huge amount of unresolved trauma in their life, guilt, shame, compulsive anger, rage, repressed hatred. It brings them some form of comfort to have the chaos in their lives and the lives of others around them. It is too painful to witness order that they cannot experience because they do not know how to create it for themselves. It takes peace of heart to create harmony and order. It is a tall order for a person with a chaotic construct to shift into orderly and serene mode.

If you encourage a toxic person to detoxify and they feel as if the detoxification process is causing them to lose their identity, they may have some deep-seated control issues. They may carry a maladaptive identity but to them, it is an identity anyway; they would rather have a maladaptive identity than no identity at all. Lots of toxic people would prefer to make do with a maladaptive identity than to adapt to a higher level of functioning whose frequency they cannot sustain. Because toxic beings have become accustomed to believe that it is too much work to be a well- rounded person, they may take the path of least resistance. Detoxification is the equivalent of wiping out dysfunctional programming to replace it with a more functional dynamic.

Toxic humans attached to dysfunction may avoid detoxification at all costs, due to a part of their program that is designed to reject a functional dynamic. They may be in certain professions or relationships that require a high level of toxicity to function. These people may be in professions such as law enforcement, correction facility management, the judiciary, drug dealing, butchering, animal slaughter, money laundering, surgery, mortuary care, etc. These people unconsciously know that detoxification is an upgrade that could cause more disturbances in their lives than they are ready to handle. They must keep running their program as toughies in order to appear authoritative and send a message that they are not to be messed with. At times, these people may resent anyone who makes them aware that detoxification is in their best interest.

With the issue of toxicity, there is always something we need to learn from the experiences of our life so we can productively move to a higher level of personal development. We can choose to look at the sum total of all the knowledge that is involved in the realm of our collective consciousness, or we can choose to look at its individual parts. One of the problems with looking at the parts is that it is mostly a left-brain activity that orients us toward a particular specialty or focus. Looking at parts also inhibits our ability to see the whole picture. The process of looking at the whole is an all-inclusive dynamic that refines our understanding, expands our sensitivities, and brings us to a higher level of mastery of the matter.

For levity:

Hank is sitting at the bar staring at his drink when a large, tattooed biker steps up next to him, grabs his drink and gulps it down in one swig. Then he shouts with his fist in Hank's face: "Well, whatcha' gonna do about it?" As Hank burst into tears the biker says: "Come on, man, I didn't think you'd cry. Dude I was just messin' with ya."

Hank keeps sobbing: "This is the worst day of my life, everything has gone wrong... This morning, I was late for a meeting so my boss fired me. When I went to the parking lot, I found that my car had been stolen and I don't have any insurance. In my turmoil, I left my wallet in the cab I took home. When I arrived home, I found my wife in bed with another man... I yelled at them and then my dog bit me. So I came to this bar to work up the courage to put an end to it all. I bought this drink I dropped a cyanide capsule in... and I've been sitting here watching the poison dissolve; the next thing I know, you show up and drink the whole damn thing! But hell, enough about me. How are you doing?"

~ Anon

Chapter 21

Maintaining the Levels of Successful Detoxification

"Much of the success of life depends upon keeping one's mind open to opportunity and seizing it when it comes."

~ Alice Foote MacDougall

Success, as anything else, requires a certain level of maintenance for its sustained continuation. This process entails the ongoing practice of healthy habits.

Keep causality in mind

Remember that every cause has an effect and that every time you operate with a negative template, you end up with negative results. The basics are simple: you are what you breathe, drink, shower with, cook with, dress with, listen to, watch, think, and participate in. Before you take an action that you either doubt or know might have some negative influence on your self, ask yourself what consequences such action may have on you one week to one year from now.

Honor and nurture the different aspects of the self daily

This may mean working on the self with the intention of achieving wholeness on all levels of one's person. It is important to include pleasant exercises that you enjoy, keeping yourself joyful, and having some form of connection with the power within you.

Do daily self-nurturing to help strengthen your:
- **Physical health**
- **Psychological health**
- **Spiritual health**

Some self-nurturing activities which are enjoyable and beneficial:

1. Go out in nature and reconnect with Earth. Observe wild life, mammals, marine animals, aquatic life, minerals, and connect with all that exists. There is so much to learn from nature and wild life. The beach, a park, a nature preserve, a natural sanctuary, any setting that is clean, features sunlight and trees, a place where to walk barefoot – such as a labyrinth -- will do. Exploring nature can be a lifelong learning experience. The infrastructure is designed for fast transportation but not for the people's enjoyment of their natural surroundings, but research sanctuaries to enjoy anyway.

2. Take a walk: it detoxifies your lymphatic system and stimulates the production of endorphins that eventually make you feel euphoric when you are done walking.

3. Do good things for other people. It enhances your self-worth.

4. Get regular professional massages or bodywork by a holistic therapist.

5. Attend spiritual gatherings with like-minded people.

6. Explore swimming with dolphins.

> *"A day spent without the sight or sound of beauty, the contemplation of mystery, or the search for truth or perfection is a poverty-stricken day, and a succession of such days is fatal to human life."*
>
> ~ Lewis Mumford (1892 - 1990)

Insist on joy

When it comes to maintaining a high level of optimism and functionality, joy is an important factor to consider developing. Keep yourself happy, rejoice, celebrate your new life and expect the best. There are various ways to make yourself happy in non-toxic ways:

1. **Explore music**: listen to music, get involved with musical instruments or musical activities. Joyful, beautiful, elevating sounds can be cathartic, therefore healing on many levels; it is one of the quickest and most non-toxic ways to create happiness for the self. Additionally, music therapy is legal, lawful, with no side effects, no risk of overdose or abuse.

2. **Seek to use humor often**. Be of good cheer and good dispositions. Our inner guidance is calling us to find our joy. Some people have had a family environment that has provided them with joy and higher expectations. For those who have not, they can benefit from creating their own space and time where they can connect

with the right sense of family. Those who have experienced a lack of nurture in their early years on this earthly plane are to work on finding their joy and healing. Our higher nature deserves to be the recipient of unlimited love. There is a time when we experience situations that echo the events of the past. We are to do everything in our power to heal the past as it usually is a perilous launching pad. When we insist on experiencing truth about ourselves and anchor it in our heart with joy, then we can experience healing.

Practice serenity

To enjoy serenity, one must first intend to experience it, then engage in doing the things that make one feel serene. This process can be the resultant of harmonious organization of ones' personal affairs, the enjoyment of a pleasant atmosphere, uplifting company, meditation, music, etc.

> *"To the mind that is still, the whole universe surrenders."*
>
> ~ Lao Tzu

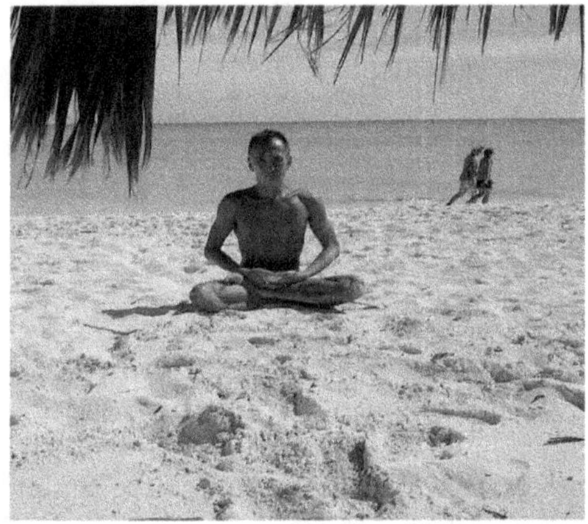

Source: commons.wikimedia.org/Wiki

Turn within

By creating time to be in the silence daily, one may discover the world within that is a source of infinite wisdom. It is in making a habit of developing right brain faculties, and balancing them out with left brain functions that one can more easily gain access to the ability to produce more neural pathways. This type of self-reliance allows you to be self-sufficient rather than counting on external sources whose moral compass may not be compatible with yours.

Meditate

Used for more than 2,500 years in the Buddhist tradition and other spiritual practices, meditation is now known in the mainstream as offering numerous benefits for the mind and body. The Boston Globe has recently reported that meditation helps reduce levels of cortisol, a stress hormone related to illness and premature aging. Meditation also helps produce more neurons that connect both hemispheres of the brain and are known to enhance the mind-body connection. Here is an inspiring and supportive article on the topic of meditation from the Boston Globe: http://www.bostonglobe.com/business/2013/04/13/meditation-can-bring-health-benefits-and-aid-function-aging-brains-research-suggests/FmMX72sGx4mIRDzxArkUaO/story.html

Practice self-discipline

There are techniques designed to promote a higher level of self-discipline. They can be explored solo or in a group, with a coach or through several media such as print, video, or audio.

Resolve to learn something constructive daily

People who immerse themselves in productive learning and the practical application of their knowledge live healthier, happier, and longer lives. You become what your mind processes and repetition always potentiates results; reinforcement is a powerful *manifestor*, whether positive or negative. Those who are addicted to bad news may want to reflect on the effects it has on the quality of their daily life. Simply ask yourself: *"Is this what I want to create in my life?"*

Find your passion

Make a list of all your goals, wishes, and desires. Choose to act on embracing the tasks that will get you to accomplish what you aim, and set a realistic deadline for their fulfillment.

Keep naysayers at bay

Those who resemble assemble, and before long become more of the same. It is best to excuse oneself from the company of naysayers whose frequency is not a vibrational match because it is not attuned to healing or purity.

"If you wish to be held in esteem,
you must associate only with those who are esteemable."

~ Jean de la Bruyere

Have a support system

When you can enjoy the company of more positive people who are capable of giving you proper validation and encouragement, it will positively reinforce the good decisions and choices you make. Toxic people will never encourage you to improve. They would be violating their own covenant to owe their allegiance to chaos. It is remarkable to see how animals have their own wisdom that can also be applied to humans. For instance, when geese fly together, they usually fly in a V formation. In this pattern, they fly 70% faster. In the event that a goose gets injured during the flight, the whole flock stops flying and stays with the injured goose until it either recovers or is laid to rest. Long-term observers of animals have found out that geese are capable of mating for life. Obviously, if there were any divorce attorneys in the world of geese, they would all starve to death. Just like geese, people usually do better on their journey when they receive selfless encouragement from supportive beings.

For levity:

The Church says: The body is a sin.
Science says: The body is a machine.
Advertising says: The body is a business.
The body says: I am a fiesta.

~ Eduardo Galeano

Conclusion

"Be the change you wish to see in the world."

~ Mahatma Gandhi

Although we live in a toxic world and the toxicity is overwhelming for all life forms, we humans must keep in mind that awareness of the issue is the first step toward solving it. An issue properly identified is one that has better chances of finding effective resolution. We can be aware of what the issues are but do not need to be consumed by the negativity that we are witnessing and experiencing. The second step is to take action and start detoxifying on all levels.

We have the prerogative to exercise choices. Some of these choices include being proactive rather than reactive, non-toxic versus toxic. We can choose to be part of the solution by doing something constructive about it or choose to remain a part of the problem by doing nothing or not helping those who are solution oriented. A cardinal rule is to not let fear dictate how to remain a part of the problem. Usually, fear activates herd instinct and irrational reactions such as insurgences. Similarly, conformity programming in fearful people may prompt a need to turn against those who are perceived as being outside of the herd. When some people feel that a problem is too insurmountable for them to handle, they may feel victimized and resort to dwelling in inertia. Inept people may feel pushed around for having to face the issue of toxicity and step out of their comfort zone. If they think that managing the toxic problem that they face or created is too big of an ordeal, they may rebel against the messenger and act antagonistic to protect their ego. Toxic people may need to protect their illusion that there is nothing to change because they believe that there is nothing wrong going on. If you think there is nothing wrong going on, check reports on whales come ashore to beach themselves due to extreme discomfort in the overly polluted ocean waters. Usually, it is the least informed people who overreact the quickest, and in the most negative of ways. Bertrand Russell, a British philosopher, has articulated this dynamic through his quote: *"The degree of one's emotions varies inversely with knowledge of facts – the less you know, the hotter you get."*

Know that when dealing with issues of toxicity, it takes discipline and discernment to focus on solutions at the elevated position of game changers. Also know that it takes mental effort and character to be proactive and optimistic when one encounters a major problem with toxicity, such as the environmental mess and weight issues. Detoxify and watch the inconvenient excess weight drop without a need to diet. It is the actions we take to troubleshoot and the optimism we generate that are likely to counteract any feeling of helplessness or victimization.

Wherever there is strife, there is likely to be toxicity. Strife, disharmony, ignorance, and a refusal to seek truth all contribute to the perpetuation of toxicity. Most of the reasons behind all that is a lack of peace, which stems from a lack of love and compassion, which both originate from a lack of awareness; a lack of awareness can also be translated as restrictive darkness associated with personal and collective ignorance. Wherever there is ignorance, there is toxicity. A simple example of that: people would not need to pass their colds or flu viruses around if they simply had the sense to wash their hands often and appropriately.

With all the health solutions that are touted in the m e d i c a l world, if the world's population is getting sicker and more overweight, then the issue is not a lack of medical products and services, but a lack of awareness of the overall issue of toxicity. Fat cells are toxic cells. If we are to stop the systematic intoxication of our body, the planet, and all that exists, we are to learn to do it with a non predatory, collaborative and peaceful mentality. The competitive mind is not always conducive to evolving in harmony. When we reach critical mass in our collaboration for solutions to the problem of toxicity, then we can reach a higher level of wellness, therefore world peace. A lack of peace leads to social unrest, illogical decisions, and assured biological obliteration. In many cases, the weapon of self-destruction or mass destruction is intoxication through foodstuff and consumer goods. We are to remember that it is the most unhappy people that are the most self-destructive and leave the most toxic pollutants in their body, their home, and the environment. Those who exhibit the most eagerness to destroy the populace, the infrastructure, and the environment are antagonistic to life itself.

> *"Let every individual and institution now think and act as a responsible trustee of Earth, seeking choices in ecology, economics and ethics that will provide a sustainable future, eliminate pollution, poverty and violence, awaken the wonder of life and foster peaceful progress in the human adventure."*
>
> ~ John McConnell, founder of International Earth Day

Just as we already know that leading by example is best, we are to set the example of detoxifying ourselves and our lives by taking action instead of watching and waiting. When it comes to detoxification choices, we can commit to making the necessary lifestyle changes that are beneficial on all levels. Such changes involve conscious detoxification and the reduction of our ecological footprint. We can also get involved in helping detoxify the planet and other people.

If one's heart is not at peace, one cannot be in harmony with nature and the cosmos. If one is not in harmony with nature and the cosmos, one can never be in harmony with the self and the world. If one is not in harmony with the self and the world, one is essentially toxic. For every problem there is a solution. By consciously working on resolution, we choose to be part of the solution rather than being part of the problem. To be part of the solution, we must take a pro-active stance as doers and be an inspiration as well as a motivating force for all other sentient beings on the planet. This stance entails working on reducing our carbon footprint to its bare minimum by diminishing toxicity through reusing and repurposing recyclable items while avoiding toxic goods. This only can ensure better health and harmony for all life forms on Earth.

HOW TO DETOXIFY YOUR LIFE NATURALLY

A complete guide to detoxification for physical, emotional, and environmental wellness

Author's biography

Sri Regine Lherisson-Bey, Ph.D. candidate, is a holistic mind-body therapist and life coach unanimously recognized as a Wellness Expert for her outstanding work with mind-body education. She is the author of the CD *Get Slim Effortlessly*. Since 1991, Therapist Lherisson-Bey has been coaching and writing about wellness and environmental awareness, with a focus on detoxification for Weight Management and Pain Control.

The author is an award-winning graduate of Saint Peter's University and a recipient of the Spur Society Award for high academic achievement and humanitarian services to the community. She has received her graduate education in Counseling Psychology at Seton Hall University. She is currently completing a doctorate degree in Integrative Medicine. Sri Regine Lherisson-Bey's professional background is in Psychology, Physiology, Biology, Nutrition, Hypnotherapy, Social and Political Sciences, Anthropology, Ethnology, and Ministerial Counseling. She has collaborated on projects ranging from medical assistance to psychophysiology research. The author advocates the preservation of indigenous cultures for the validation of ancient natural therapies.

For over two decades, Sri Regine Lherisson-Bey's articles on wellness and environmental awareness have been published in various holistic magazines nationwide. The author has been an invited guest on several radio and television programs featuring her work on wellness for the mind and body.

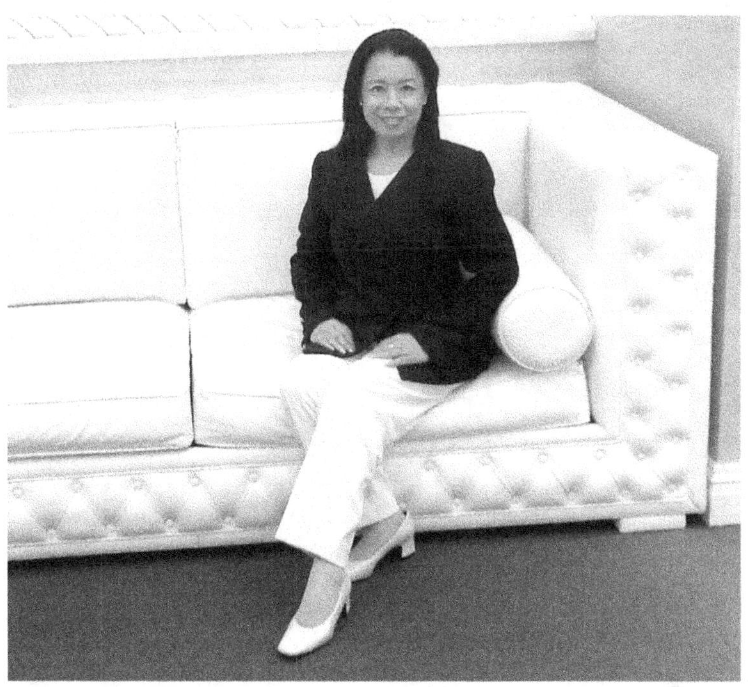

http://www.howtodetoxifyyourlifenaturally.com